Medicine *Culture*

Varieties
of Treatment in the
United States, England,
West Germany, and France

Lynn Payer

A Holt Paperback
Henry Holt and Company
New York

Holt Paperbacks
Henry Holt and Company, LLC
Publishers since 1866
175 Fifth Avenue
New York, New York 10010
www.henryholt.com

A Holt Paperback® and ® are registered trademarks of
Henry Holt and Company, LLC.

Library of Congress Cataloging-in-Publication Data
Payer, Lynn.
Medicine and culture: varieties of treatment in the
United States, England, West Germany, and France/
Lynn Payer.—1st Holt Paperbacks ed.
p.   cm.
"Originally published in hardcover in 1988 by
Henry Holt and Company"—CIP t.p. verso.
Includes bibliographical references and index.
ISBN-13: 978-0-8050-4803-2

1. Social medicine—Europe.   2. Social medicine—United States.
3. Physician and patient—Europe.   4. Physician and patient—
United States.   I. Title.
RA418.3.E85P39   1996   96-27481
610'.94—dc20   CIP

Henry Holt books are available for special promotions and
premiums. For details contact: Director, Special Markets.

Originally published in hardcover in 1988 by
Henry Holt and Company

First Holt Paperbacks Edition 1996

Designed by Ann Gold

Printed in the United States of America

D 20 19 18 17

Medicine & Culture

This book is dedicated to the memory of my mother, whose English ancestry may explain her tendency to greet new scientific developments with a skeptical ''How do they know that?'' It is also dedicated to my father, whose French ancestry may explain his proclivity to halve the doses of medicine prescribed for him.

Contents

Foreword to the
Owl Books Edition
The More Things Change . . .

Eight years have passed since *Medicine and Culture* first appeared, and those eight years have seen dramatic changes in both the world at large and the world of medicine. Consider just two developments affecting the four countries examined in *Medicine and Culture*: the Wall between West and East Germany has literally disappeared, and 1992 marked the year when the walls blocking commerce were supposed to disappear between the countries of the European Community.

In the world of medicine, much has also changed. Alternative medicine has become much more popular with patients in the United States, and it is no longer uncommon for Americans, at least in New York City and California, to talk about their homeopathic or herbal remedies or their appointments with their acupuncturist. Women with breast cancer in the United States, at least those living in some areas, now have a chance of being offered a treatment that conserves their breasts. Nutrition guidelines published in 1995 actually told Americans that a little bit of wine might be good for their health. The United States has debated and rejected health care reform and ultimately ended up with a new nonsystem, one that has changed the incentives in

xii   Foreword to the Owl Books Edition

our country from doing too much to patients to, in some cases, doing too little. The spread of acquired immunodeficiency syndrome (AIDS) throughout the world has shattered our optimism about medicine's ability to conquer disease as well as underlined the importance of the immune system in keeping us healthy. And the movement known as evidence-based medicine is making heroic efforts to improve the science base of clinical medicine, to help ensure that medicine does more good than harm to patients.

But the way these particular changes have occurred only underscores the important role that national cultures play in medical practice:

- Prior to the fall of the Wall, German medicine could be divided into two distinct cultures. While both East and West Germany shared a common heritage of medical practice up to World War II, the two separate states formed after the war took very divergent pathways on some issues, notably on alternative medicines. East German government policy discouraged their use and even outlawed some medical systems, including homeopathy. West German government policy, by contrast, encouraged the sale of many different kinds of remedies. This protection of alternative medicine occurred even when regulatory authorities tried to ban certain substances they believed dangerous or ineffective: the West German courts ruled in favor of the substances and those who were selling them. Now, of course, the cultures are merging, with the former Western culture becoming the dominant culture of Germany in medicine as well as in everything else. Homeopathic and other alternative medicines are now legal throughout reunited Germany.
- The common market in pharmaceutical products has begun, but much more slowly than predicted. Initially set for 1992, in that year not one pharmaceutical preparation had been authorized for sale in all the countries of the European Community. Representatives of the various countries could not agree on which drugs should be readily available because they were weighing the risks and benefits quite differently: French dele-

gates, I was told, were more concerned about the toxic effects of drugs on the liver than were their colleagues in other countries of the EC. When delegates realized that there was no way that each country was going to accept the decisions of other countries as to what products to allow on the market, they sought another solution. Currently, each country in the European Community retains its barriers to products from the others, although pharmaceutical companies may now apply to a commission in Great Britain to register their products in all the countries simultaneously. By late 1995, the commission had registered exactly one drug.

• Alternative medicine is becoming more popular with patients in the United States, but it's still much less common than in Western Europe. While one study showed that about one-third of U.S. residents reached by telephone had used some form of alternative medicine during the preceding twelve months, this figure included those who had used relaxation or massage therapies or who had participated in a commercial diet program or a self-help group, which would all be considered mainstream in many other countries. Only 1 percent reported having used homeopathy in the past twelve months, and 3 percent herbal medicines. In France, by contrast, 36 percent of the population reported using homeopathy in 1992, up from 16 percent in 1982.

• Women found to have breast cancer in the United States *may* now be offered a lumpectomy, depending on where they live, but many women and their doctors continue to choose radical mastectomy. While the majority of women with breast cancer can be safely treated by a lumpectomy, an analysis of 1993 Medicare data showed that in some areas of the country lumpectomies were performed on only 1.4 percent of women with breast cancer. In the areas of the country with the highest uses of lumpectomy, still under half of women with breast cancer received this operation, although about 80 percent were eligible.

Interestingly, when journalists discovered that one investigator in a lumpectomy versus mastectomy study had lied about
some patients' results, skewing his outcome in favor of lumpectomies, American reporters responded by showing their bias
for studies performed in the United States. Even if the falsified
data entered by the one investigator *had* altered the U.S.
study's conclusions (and since his patients accounted for only a
fraction of the total, even if he'd changed all his bad results to
good ones the final data weren't going to be much different), a
number of earlier lumpectomy trials in Europe strongly indicated that this operation was as safe for most women as a mastectomy. It was highly unlikely that the conclusions of the U.S.
study would have changed much, however fraudulent the
data—and, in my opinion, the press needlessly worried women
about the operation in the face of so much other evidence.

- While Americans are now prescribed a little bit of wine for
  their health (why does no one say for their enjoyment?), pregnant women, or even women of childbearing age, are told they
  should not drink at all, despite the fact that there's little evidence that occasional or even moderate drinking is harmful to
  the fetus. When, in 1994, I asked a French doctor in charge of
  public health campaigns what advice was given to pregnant
  French women about drinking, he looked surprised. None, he
  said, since the issue was simply not considered important.

- During the debate over health care reform in the United States,
  the arguments most commonly cited to discredit the single-
  payer Canadian system were those of the relatively small number of CAT scanners and MRIs available in Canada, and the
  supposedly long waiting lists for elective procedures. Nobody
  was able to argue convincingly that Canadian health suffered
  overall from a lack of either technology, since Canadians spend
  less on health care and live longer than U.S. citizens do. But in
  the United States, where many people assume that good medicine consists of doing as many high-tech tests as quickly as possible, it was simply assumed that there were serious deficien-
  cies in the Canadian system.

With the debate over health care reform now a memory, the United States is currently caught in a battle between conflicting culture values. We've always valued doing things to patients, preferably as much as possible. But we also have a mystical belief in the wisdom of the market to meet needs of whatever sort. In the past, the two values often dovetailed, with market forces pushing toward more and more procedures. But the steep increase in health care costs has caused a reorganization of the market. When health care providers get paid per patient, rather than per act, the financial incentive is to do as little as possible, thus putting the providers in direct conflict with what patients have been conditioned to expect.

While the new economic incentives in health care may, over the years, change the American patients' expectations for aggressive treatment, their preferences for more, and more intense, treatment remain strong, particularly when compared to that of British doctors and patients. A study that came out in the fall of 1988 showed how great this divide really was. British, Canadian, and American specialists in genitourinary oncology were asked how they personally would want to be treated if they had certain cancers. For locally advanced bladder cancer, 92 percent of American and Canadian specialists wanted radical surgery, compared to only 30 percent of British specialists. In the case of localized prostate cancer, 79 percent of the American specialists, 61 percent of the Canadian specialists, and only 4 percent of the British specialists wanted radical surgery. I am often asked whether the British preference for doing as little as possible simply reflects the economics of the National Health Service. Deciding how much to pay for what procedures is certainly a reflection of how a culture values those procedures, but this study proved to my satisfaction that values played a role above and beyond economic considerations.

Both the aggressive American approach to medicine and the conservative British approach are enforced by the courts in their respective countries. In 1992, an American court ruled that hospitals must continue to treat an infant with no brain if the parents want treatment; in the same year a British court ruled the opposite.

These preferences are also reflected in the way the two nations have adopted new treatments or gotten rid of old ones. Americans still like to treat until treatment has been shown to be harmful; British doctors like to wait until treatment has proven beneficial, and then they're likely to ask, How beneficial? While American doctors began treating mild cardiac arrythmias with anti-arrythmic drugs until a study found that at least two of the drugs used were killing patients, the British didn't have to change their practice as a result of the study because they hadn't been treating as such this particular group of patients. When an American study concluded that AIDS patients who were given AZT showed improvement in their T-cell counts, American doctors claimed that all patients with AIDS should be treated with AZT. The British demurred, waiting for an endpoint more significant than improved blood counts, and when the final results were in the British were largely correct: AZT didn't really prolong life, but simply corrected the blood counts. American doctors now believe that giving AZT to pregnant women who are HIV positive can reduce the risk of their transmitting the virus to their babies: again, British doctors are not yet convinced, calling the results too few and too preliminary.

As I wrote in 1988, patients and doctors in England and America, while often taking opposite sides on the issue of whether it is better to do something or do nothing, tend to see disease as something that comes from the outside. By contrast, Continental doctors and patients are more likely to emphasize weaknesses of particular organs or imbalances between various organs and/or systems. I was startled to learn a few years ago that the French have no phrase comparable to the "germ theory of disease." They talk instead about the germ theory of *transmissible* disease, a much more limited role for germs in the scheme of things.

AIDS has caused us to consider these two metaphors of disease causation simultaneously: the AIDS virus comes from outside the body and attacks, yet it has made Americans more aware of the crucial role that internal defenses play in keeping one healthy. Perhaps as a result, Americans have begun to take tonics and immune system stimulants just as Europeans have done for years. Interestingly, one study showed that French doctors are less afraid of treating people with AIDS than are Canadian and American doctors, perhaps partly due to the fact that they aren't as afraid of catching the virus in the course of general medical care, and partly due to their less puritanical view of people with a disease transmitted most commonly through sexual contact.

But while AIDS has made us more aware of the crucial role of the immune system in fighting disease, the idea of diseases that attack from the outside is still strong in England and America. I once overheard a Frenchman say that the only thing Americans fear are germs and communists, and with the collapse of Eastern European communism, the fear of germs seems to be getting stronger. Certainly, new infectious diseases continue to be identified, and AIDS is an example of one that is serious and widespread. But the press in both Britain and the United States continues to get overly excited about other diseases that are neither new nor particularly on the rise. The best example occurred when streptococcus A, the flesh-eating bacteria, made the headlines, first in Great Britain and later in the United States. This disease, while certainly horrendous for those suffering from it, had been around for a long time, and there was no good evidence that it was increasing. Was the public and media's concern over this disease a sign that, in the absence of the Red menace, and a bit weary from AIDS, we needed new enemies to worry about?

One of the most fascinating developments to occur since 1988 has been the interplay of the common explanatory models for fatigue. As I wrote in the first editon of *Medicine and Culture*, French doctors will diagnose vague symptoms as spasmophilia or something to do with the liver; German doctors will explain it as due to the heart, low blood pressure, or vasovegetative dystonia; the British will see it as a mood disorder such as depression; and Americans are likely to search for a viral or allergic cause. Not too long after *Medicine and Culture* came out, a British psychiatrist, Dr.

Simon Wessely, decided to look at the evidence for the German belief that low blood pressure and fatigue are correlated. To his surprise, they were: British patients with low blood pressure (who didn't necessarily know they had it) indeed reported that they were more tired than the average patient. (Dr. Wessely's study, published in the *British Medical Journal*, came to the typically British conclusion that there was no particular reason to treat low blood pressure even if it was associated with fatigue, perhaps a sign that the work ethic has never been that strong in Great Britain.) More recently, American researchers found that American patients diagnosed with chronic fatigue syndrome had an abnormal blood pressure response when they were turned upside down, another piece of the puzzle indicating that the German explanation of fatigue as a circulatory problem may be nearer to the underlying physiology in many patients than the infectious explanations favored in the United States. I'm convinced that a man I know who keeps fainting would be better off if American doctors recognized the German concept of circulatory collapse.

Finally, there has been a much greater effort to find out which medicines really work, and a movement to try to use only those therapies that do more good than harm. A movement known as evidence-based medicine is growing, with the most visible hallmark being the Cochrane Collaboration based in Oxford, England. The Cochrane Collaboration is named after Dr. Archibald Cochrane, who is quoted in my chapter on culture bias in medical science about what a map of the world would look like if colored according to the number of randomized, controlled clinical trials carried out in individual countries. In his classic 1971 book *Effectiveness and Efficiency*, Dr. Cochrane wrote that if black indicated the highest number, then "one would see the UK in black and scattered black patches in Scandinavia, the USA and a few other countries: The rest would be nearly white." Surely that map today would be much blacker everywhere than it was at that time. But while nearly everyone today accepts the randomized, controlled trial as the gold standard for clinical research, there are still cultural differences in the way such trials are carried out: the devil is in the details. Countries such as the United States, where doctors and patients still believe that it's always better to do something rather than nothing, will decide that it's unethical to have a placebo arm; end the trial sooner; or find some ways to get around the process of randomization. A researcher conducting a randomized trial to see if bone-marrow transplants prolong the life of patients with breast cancer had trouble recruiting enough patients because they feared being randomized into the arm of the trial that did not include a bone-marrow transplant, showing that women in the United States still believe that doing something is always better than doing nothing, even if you don't know if the something works.

And while the science of clinical trials has advanced, whether the science ultimately gets translated into patient care is another matter entirely. Nowhere is this more evident than in the recommendations concerning the age at which regular mammographic screening for breast cancer should start. Most European countries recommend starting at age fifty, since the more rigorous studies of mammography in women below that age consistently show that the death rates from breast cancer in women who are screened are at least as high as in women of comparable risk who are not. After a Canadian study showed that the death rate might even be higher in young women who were screened, the National Cancer Institute dropped its recommendation that women under fifty have regular mammograms. This caused an intense outcry: a congressional committee convened to investigate the NCI committee that had lifted its recommendation, criticizing it for, among other things, relying too heavily on data obtained from tests on foreign women (even though the most rigorous trials had been done on foreign women). The American College of Radiology continues to issue regular press releases that support screening for younger women, in marked contrast to the Royal College of Radiology in Britain, which warns women away from unnecessary mammograms.

In his foreword to *Medicine and Culture* in 1988, Dr. Kerr White estimated that only 15 percent of medicine was based on science, that is, on objective evidence that the intervention would do the patient more good than harm. Dr. White thinks that today the situation is slightly better, and he would hazard that the overall figure might be 20 to 25 percent. Of course, the figure varies greatly depending on the country, the institution, and the doctor.

I have two regrets about the original edition of *Medicine and Culture*. One is that I did not discuss the role of religion in the United States, where it has obvious and direct effects on the practice of medicine. The other is that I used the term "national character." While I think it possible that "national character" does exist, the concept was not really necessary to explain the medical differences I detailed. National culture is sufficient, and I think my description of what I meant by national character makes it plain that I meant the effect of national culture on the people who grow up in that culture. The term national character offends many people, and there's no need to invoke it when culture explains so much.

Finally, I'd like to correct one impression that some readers had from *Medicine and Culture*. Leaders in the battle for health care reform in the United States told me that representatives of the American Medical Association would say "it will never work in the United States," waving copies of *Medicine and Culture* in support of their position.

I hope that acknowledging the role that culture plays in medicine does not become an excuse for fatalism, such as "ethnic tensions" often becomes in international affairs. As an American, I do believe that you can change things. But I think that you can change them more effectively if you understand the culture you're up against. And I still think that in no other area is this truer than in medicine.

Lynn Payer
New York, 1996

A note about references: many readers of the 1988 edition of Medicine and Culture *complained that they weren't aware of my extensive references at the back until they had finished the book. Publishers of trade books don't like to clutter the text with little superscript numbers, so a common way to include references is to put them at the back, keying them to the first words of a paragraph. If you want to find the source of any of my assertions, note the page number and the first words of the paragraph, and look it up in the back section. This does not hold true, however, for references to the foreword to the Owl Books edition. These follow here:*

Page

xii Prior to the fall of the Wall: Peter Fisher and Adam Ward, "Complementary Medicine in Europe," *British Medical Journal* 309 (July 9, 1994):107–10; "Germany: Court Order Responsible for Fatal Events?" *The Lancet* 340 (July 11, 1992):107–108.

xiii Alternative medicine is becoming more popular: David M. Eisenberg et al., "Unconventional Medicine in the United States," *The New England Journal of Medicine* 328 (1993):246–52.

xiii Women found to have breast cancer in the United States: DeAnn Lazovich et al., "Underutilization of Breast-Conserving Surgery and Radiation Therapy Among Women with Stage I or II Breast Cancer," *Journal of the American Medical Association* 266 (Dec. 25, 1991):3433–38; Gina Kolata, "Sharp Regional Incongruity Found in Medical Costs and Treatments: Surgery for Breast Cancer Shows Most Extreme Variation," *The New York Times*, Jan. 30, 1996, C3.

xv With the debate over health care reform now a memory: Charles Hampden-Turner and Fons Trompenaars, *The Seven Cultures of Capitalism* (New York: Doubleday, 1993).

xv While the new economic incentives in health care: Malcom J. Moore, Brian O'Sullivan, and Ian F. Tannock, "How Expert Physicians Would Wish to Be Treated If They Had Genitourinary Cancer," *Journal of Clinical Oncology* 6 (Nov. 1988):1736–45.

xv Both the aggressive American approach to medicine: Frances Miller, "Infant Resuscitation, a US/UK Divide," *The Lancet* 343 (June 25, 1994):1584–85.

xvi These preferences are also reflected in: Thomas J. Moore, *Deadly Medicine: Why Tens of Thousands of Heart Patients Died in America's Worst Drug Disaster* (New York: Simon & Schuster, 1995); John D. Hamilton et al., "A Controlled Trial of Early Versus Late Treatment with Zidovudine in

Symptomatic Human Immunodeficiency Virus Infection," *The New England Journal of Medicine* 326 (Feb. 13, 1992):437–43; "Zidovudine for Mother, Fetus, and Child: Hope or Poison?" *The Lancet* 344 (July 23, 1994):207–9.

xvi   AIDS has caused us to consider these two metaphors: Martin F. Shapiro et al., "Residents' Experiences in, and Attitudes Toward, the Care of Persons with AIDS in Canada, France, and the United States," *Journal of the American Medical Association* 268 (July 22/29, 1992):510–15.

xvii   But while AIDS: "Flesh-Eating Virus Invades the U.S.: No American Is Safe, Says Centers for Disease Control," cover of *Weekly World News*, June 28, 1994; Laurie Garrett, "How Bad Is Bug? Docs Differ on Flesh-Eating Strep's Potential Threat to Public Health," *New York Newsday*, June 10, 1994, A20.

xvii   One of the most fascinating developments: Simon Wessely et al., "Symptoms of Low Blood Pressure: A Population Study," *British Medical Journal* 301 (1990):362–65; Issam Bou-Holaigah et al., "The Relationship Between Neurally Medicated Hypotension and the Chronic Fatigue Syndrome," *Journal of the American Medical Association* 274 (Sept. 27, 1995):961–67; Hugh Calkins et al., "The Economic Burden of Unrecognized Vasodepressor Syncope," *The American Journal of Medicine* 95 (Nov. 1993):473–79.

xviii Finally, there has been a much greater effort: Kenneth F. Schulz, "Subverting Randomization in Controlled Trials," *Journal of the American Medical Association* 274 (Nov. 8, 1995):1456–58; Gina Kolata, "Women Rejecting Trials for Testing a Cancer Therapy," *The New York Times*, Feb. 15, 1995, 1.

xix   And while the science of clinical trials: Committee on Government Operations, "Misused Science: The National Cancer Institute's Elimination of Mammography Guidelines for Women in Their Forties" (U.S. Government Printing Office: Washington, D.C., 1994); "Warning on Unnecessary Breast X-Ray Examinations," *British Medical Journal* 306 (Apr. 10, 1993):950.

Foreword

Three elements characterize the essence of the clinical transaction between patient and physician: technology, caring, and values. Although the nature, quality, and mix of the three vary widely in differing circumstances, each is usually present. This important volume by a seasoned medical journalist deals primarily with values, the most neglected of the three elements. For in the final analysis, it is values, both individual and collective, both the people's and the profession's, that govern the character and quality of the clinical encounter on the personal level, and the social contract on the political level. If at times the individual seems powerless in confronting a physician, we should all recall that it is society's values which ultimately determine the rights, privileges, obligations, and perquisites of the health care establishment. This book is about the widely differing, and often antagonistic, values that govern both the negotiation and the content of individual and societal transactions with the medical professions of four similarly developed Western industrialized democracies.

Perhaps values would be of less importance if there were indisputable evidence that all interventions of all physicians were always of clear benefit to all patients. Incompetence and malpractice apart, such an idyllic state of affairs lies in some remote and improbable future. Although things are much better than they were a generation ago, it is still the case that only about 15 percent of all contemporary clinical interventions are supported by objective scientific evidence that they do more good than harm. On the other hand, between 40 and 60 percent of all therapeutic benefits can be attributed to a combination of the placebo and Hawthorne effects, two code words for caring and concern, or what most people call "love." Although the placebo effect is usually dismissed as a "residual" outcome, and the Hawthorne effect as an inconsequential phenomenon restricted to industrial settings, these two ubiquitous responses still constitute the most powerful, all-purpose, therapeutic interventions available to the profession. Surely their influence is at least one plausible explanation for the apparently favorable results associated with the wide range of medical maneuvers employed for seemingly similar sets of symptoms and disorders brought to physicians in the diverse settings examined in this volume.

But what of values? Here Lynn Payer has provided us with a vivid synthesis of statistics, critical observations, and lively anecdotes that document the differing value systems of the four countries—countries that have much in common but quite different cultures, views of the human condition, concepts of health and disease, and approaches to medical practice. Payer provides chapter and verse at both the macro and micro levels to make the case that differences in national character and professional responses to patients' problems are important determinants of clinical care. International comparisons that emphasize values, underlying paradigms, and outcomes of care may well yield greater understanding of the optimal ways in which to improve health and ameliorate disease than traditional comparisons restricted to measures of facilities, manpower, use, and costs.

Indeed, such are the tenuous links between what physicians do technically in the process of treating patients and the outcomes of that care that even demonstrably efficacious interventions vary widely in their practical effectiveness in diverse settings. Miscommunication, noncompliance, different concepts of the nature of illness and what to do about it, and, above all, different values and preferences of patients and their physicians limit the potential benefits of both technology and caring.

How did the medical profession ever develop the notion that its values should take precedence over those of patients and the public? Given the profession's long track record of error, and its brief history of seemingly rational medicine, largely the fruits of advances in the fundamental sciences, why should such insensitivity persist? The usual explanation is the public's propensity for endowing the medical profession with priestly, and in some cultures, paternalistic, attributes that encourages many of its members to make unquestioned, and too often unsubstantiated, authoritarian pronouncements in private and in public on health, disease, and what is good for patients. That may be so. In the United States, however, I believe Lynn Payer is correct in suggesting another hypothesis. She ascribes the "aggressivity" of American medicine to its dominance by physicians with a strong streak, and often a hard core, of obsessive compulsive behavioral characteristics. This sort of behavior, it is said, tends to substitute activity for reflection and to confuse actions with accomplishments. Too often it may mask the physician's underlying anxiety and relative impotence to deal with the open-ended, frequently insoluble, problems of life, living, and death that are brought to physicians by their expectant patients.

"Problems that have solutions are not problems," said John Updike. Why "do something" when comforting and caring are needed and, when there is no clearly beneficial technology, more fundamental research is the best approach. As with American medicine's therapeutic endeavors, so with its aggressive approach to diagnosing. "A normal person is someone who has not been thoroughly investigated in a university hospital," goes one definition bandied about in the country's medical schools. Such misplaced curiosity wastes billions of dollars annually. This money could be applied more usefully not only to fundamental biological and behavioral research but to more research into values and value systems, and into concepts of health, disease, suffering, and death in diverse cultures. We need more transcultural studies of the type Payer has given us in this fascinating volume.

"When the patient and the physician agree on the nature of the problem, the patient gets better," said Adolf Meyer, first professor of psychiatry at the Johns Hopkins University. The analyses presented in this volume of patients' interactions with their physicians in France, Germany, the United Kingdom, and the United States affirm the underlying force of Meyer's aphorism. Lynn Payer has written a book that should appeal both to a concerned public beset by rising health care costs and an increasingly remote and mechanistic approach to medical care in America, and to a beleaguered and bewildered medical profession trying to rethink its mission and its mandate. There is indeed much to stimulate public and professional discussion in this seminal work.

Kerr L. White, M.D.
Retired Deputy Director for Health Sciences
Rockefeller Foundation

Medicine & Culture

Is Medicine International?

It is true that in his sanctum sanctorum—that secret place of his heart where he keeps his most sacred prejudices—the reader may treasure the unavowed belief that an American is superior to an Italian. He is entitled to his prejudice. And I respect it. I even think it may be useful in order to counterbalance the prejudice which the Italian no doubt treasures to the effect that he is superior to the American. All that kind of thing keeps the world going and there is not too much harm in it, provided prejudices—like dogs—are trained to behave.

—Salvador de Madariaga, *Americans*

While living in Europe and working there as a medical journalist, I was struck by the differences between U.S. and European medicine. Why, for example, did the French talk about their livers all the time? Why did the Germans blame their hearts for their fatigue when there didn't seem to be anything seriously wrong with them? Why did the British operate so much less than the Americans? And why did my French friends become upset when I said I had a virus?

At first, I was inclined to attribute all deviations from the American norm to the fact that European doctors were less well educated than those in the United States, that their medicine was more "primitive." As an American with a background in biochemistry, I believed medicine to be a science, with a "right" and "wrong" way to treat a disease, and any deviation from the American norm to be "wrong."

This view became difficult to reconcile, however, with statistics showing that Europeans have at least the same life expectancy as Americans, and in the case of some European countries a longer life expectancy. Moreover, a number of practices that I first encountered in Europe have since been adopted in the United States.

As a medical writer covering medicine in Europe for *The Medical Post* of Canada, the *International Herald Tribune*, the *Journal of the Addiction Research Foundation* of Ontario, *Medical Tribune*, *Medical World News*, *Rheumatology News*, *Oncology News*, and a number of other publications, I was in a reasonably good position to explore these differences. Whenever I encountered one, I asked, Why? This book is based on the responses I received from doctors, medical historians, and other medical observers.

As my understanding of European medical practices grew, I began to appreciate their usefulness and validity. Ways of looking at and treating illness that had at first seemed folkloric started to seem reasonable and even desirable. At the same time, I began to look at American medicine differently. Many of the practices I had taken for granted now seemed to be not so much the result of scientific progress but rather outgrowths of American cultural biases that in some cases harmed more than helped our health and well-being. In seeing how another country's cultural prejudices affected its medicine, I found it easier to perceive how our own prejudices affect our practice of medicine.

Documenting these different practices, let alone understanding their significance, has not been nearly as easy as I originally imagined. In many cases, there is no data on how common various procedures are within a country, let alone international comparisons. For example, while overall surgical statistics for the United States exist, the only statistics available in France concern data taken on one day every four years or so, called the *Journée du K*. West Germany has statistics concerning procedures done in doctors' offices, but has not kept statistics concerning hospital practices. In Britain, the organization of the

British National Health Service so simplifies the work of doctors that they need not fill out forms for everything they do; as a result, they do not have the data base that exists in some other countries.

Even when comparative studies exist, their authors often demonstrate an ignorance of basic medical practices and beliefs in the countries studied, an ignorance that limits their ability to interpret the results. One author, for example, who had compared intensive care units in France and the United States and found the death rate due to gastrointestinal problems higher in France was unaware that the French attribute many diseases to the liver and had until recently a high consumption of gastrointestinal drugs, something that anyone who has lived in France or even reads French novels would know. Another, who had compared how nurses from different cultures perceive pain in certain conditions and during various procedures, hadn't considered that in some countries the procedures would be done with anesthesia whereas in others they would not. Even doctors working with such international organizations as the World Health Organization seemed to be ignorant of large differences in medical practice among member countries. One World Health Organization doctor, for example, thought that a D & C—the third most common medical procedure in the United States— was only a euphemism for abortion; his misconception reflected his having received his medical training in France, where diagnostic D & C's are rarely performed in young women. The U.S. Center for Health Statistics offers a full range of American medical statistics, but has little data on medical practice abroad, in spite of the fact that it is the U.S. center for the International Classification of Diseases.

While I have drawn heavily on those facts that are available from both comparative and national studies, I found that I learned the most from my interviews with medical people in the various countries, who tried to explain the reasons behind the facts. The facts by themselves can be explained away as artifacts (and often are); the reasoning makes clear that the differences are real, explains why they exist—and should allow the prediction of future differences.

Originally, I gathered information on health practices in a number of European countries. Eventually, I decided to focus on three European countries and one North American one— France, West Germany, Great Britain, and the United States— for several reasons. First, these four countries represent the four predominant traditions of Western medicine and as such have an influence far beyond their respective borders. French medicine, for example, has been a leading light in the Latin countries of Italy and Spain and therefore has also been extremely influential in Latin American medicine. West German medicine represents a whole tradition of middle European medicine that reaches from Alsace to Russia and strongly influenced the development of medicine in the United States and Japan. Western medicine on the African continent derives from either English or French medicine. English and German medicine have strongly influenced Scandinavian medicine, which has produced some of the finest survival statistics in the world. In recent years, U.S. medicine, most strongly influenced by English and German medicine, has itself become extremely influential.

The four countries were also chosen because certain key statistics—infant and maternal mortality and life expectancy—were roughly equivalent in all four, which allowed me to assume that at least in terms of measurability, their medicine could be judged to be equal. The three European countries, as an added advantage, have similar populations and similar age structures, with the average age in all three being somewhat higher than in the United States.

Finally, as an American of French, German, and English ancestry who had acquired some general knowledge of French and German language and culture, I felt that my background would help me explore these particular medical cultures.

For the most part, I have tried to limit my inquiry to "legitimate medicine," i.e., that practiced or directed by persons who have the M.D. or an equivalent degree. Physicians may object when I write about homeopathy and other systems that in the United States would be judged "fringe medicine." But the fact is that most practitioners of homeopathy in Europe receive an M.D. degree before they study homeopathy, and it is impossible to write about European medicine and exclude them. Many physicians believe the only medicine worth writing about is the highly scientific medicine sometimes practiced in university hospitals, but such medicine is in fact the exception rather than the rule. Most of our encounters with the doctor are about everyday problems such as fatigue, panic attacks, high blood pressure, vaginal infections, and birth control that don't always have "scientific" solutions. The way the doctor treats such problems is often of more importance to us in our everyday lives than the perhaps more scientific and internationally standardized treatment of rare diseases.

My method has been that of a journalist, not a social scientist. As a consequence, while I have tried to interview roughly equivalent numbers of doctors in the four countries under study, I did not make numerical equivalence a priority. As a journalist, I have been suspicious of information coming from one source if it did not correlate with what I learned from others or was not backed up by credible statistical data, and I have discarded anecdotal information unless it illuminated either a statistic or a fairly widespread belief or practice.

While the material I provide on the large differences that exist in the medicine practiced in the four countries is based on fact, the reasons I offer for the differences can only be speculative. "You can never prove anything in the social sciences," I was told early on in my research for this book. Thus, while I can unearth data that clearly show that Germans use an enormous quantity of heart drugs, and I can establish with reasonable certainty on the basis of medical data that they diagnose *Herzinsuffizienz* on grounds that would not lead to a heart diagnosis in France, England, or America, my explanation that this may be due to German romanticism is speculation based on what German doctors suggested. After nine years of research,

I am convinced that it is as reasonable an explanation as any other; the reader can draw his or her own conclusions.

My search for explanations has sometimes led me to that of "national character." I realize that there are dangers in this concept, and I recognize that national stereotypes sometimes betray more about the person who holds them than about the nation, but there are also pitfalls in assuming that there is no such thing as national character. Most Americans, and probably most people of other nationalities, tend to assume as I originally did that any deviations from what they perceive as the medical norm occur only because other countries lack the resources, the organization, or the will to do as we do. This view assumes that everyone is working toward the same goals, with some countries more successful than others. But while the goals might be the same if everyone had unlimited resources, in the real world priorities must be established and they are not always the same. The English, for example, have less money to spend on health, but they nevertheless are spending what they do have quite differently than we do in America. There are only one hundred cardiologists in the whole of England—but also one hundred geriatric psychiatrists. If the English had more money, they might well spend it on the training of more geriatric psychiatrists, because to them the quality of life in old age takes precedence over preventing heart attacks.

At times, this book may appear to be overly critical, with a focus on the bizarre "different" practices of each country and a neglect of practices that are both of unquestionable value and universally practiced. There is, of course, a great deal that is similar in the medicine of the four countries under consideration, although not nearly so much as many writers would have us believe. But to study the similarities teaches us little, while exploring the differences can, I believe, teach us much. The reader should, however, keep in mind that my focus distorts the picture to some extent and that I am not attempting a comprehensive study of everything about the medicine of each country, which would make for boring reading. I recognize that I have to some extent caricaturized the doctors of each country and their medicine—not all French doctors are Cartesian, not all German doctors authoritarian romantics, not all English doctors kindly but paternalistic, not all American doctors aggressive. As with most caricatures, these pictures may be distorted, but they are based on truths found in the overall practices of each country.

While I do believe in the concept of national character, I do not believe that it is due to something immutable written in our genes but rather is a conglomeration of values, priorities, and actions that changes over time, albeit slowly. Someone who has grown up being told to think like Descartes is going to grow up thinking differently from someone who has been taught to distrust theory and pay attention only to "the facts." Someone who grew up hearing *The Little Engine That Could* every Saturday morning will see possibility in a different light from someone taught to obey at any cost. As Robert Darnton wrote in his introduction to *The Great Cat Massacre and Other Episodes in French Cultural History*: "One thing seems clear to everyone who returns from field work: other people are other. They do not think the way we do."

This otherness should be respected, not denied. In medicine, as in other fields, it shows us new possibilities for ourselves— something I discovered when I developed a medical condition that proved to elicit a number of culture biases in diagnosis and treatment.

My original interest in the subject of medical differences had been purely an intellectual one. But shortly after I had begun my research, a routine gynecologic checkup in France revealed a grapefruit-sized fibroid tumor in my uterus, a very common condition of women. While I rejected the suggestion of a colleague to become a sort of "traveling tumor," visiting doctors in a number of different countries to see what their treatment recommendations were (I don't like to see doctors any more than most people, and for my experience to have any value I would have had to see at least several doctors in each country), a recurrence of the fibroids after their initial removal by myomectomy after I had moved back to America gave me a chance to compare those two countries. In France, where great value is put on the woman's ability to bear children, hysterectomy was not even suggested as an option. Instead, the French surgeon told me I *must* have myomectomy, a major operation in which the fibroid tumor is removed while the ability to have children is preserved. I was told that six such operations could be performed without even necessitating a cesarean section were I to become pregnant. In the United States, I was put under a great deal of pressure for hysterectomy and told that a second myomectomy would be impossible. In neither case did the doctors seem to realize that their therapeutic recommendations were influenced less by the facts of my case than by how much the culture in which they operated valued the ability to have children.

However, the research and thinking I had done for this book put me in a particularly strong position to deal with these doctors. If they were not capable of separating fact from cultural bias, I was; and while I valued their facts and skills I felt their opinions were inherently no better than mine. Since it was my body, my opinions were in fact better. I pointed this out, and both ultimately agreed. As a consequence, both in France and in the United States I was able to chose a treatment, myomectomy, that best served me.

I should perhaps warn my readers that I have come up with no secret "miracle cures" for any diseases. What I think I have discovered is that the range of "acceptable" treatments for most diseases is much wider than that admitted in any one country, and a wider view of such acceptable treatments would better serve both doctors and patients. I also hope I have shown how our medical biases cause us to accept certain treatments and reject others, or to accept some too quickly and others not quickly enough. A better understanding of these biases should help to illuminate our past mistakes—and perhaps avoid future ones.

Culture Bias in
Medical Science

You will find that on one side of a frontier cellulitis means muscular rheumatism, and on the other it involves purulent inflammation of the subcutaneous tissue; a hundred kilometers further on it is a euphemism for obesity in puffy young women.
—Dr. M. N. G. Dukes

The literature shows that there are no consistent criteria even for determining body height and weight. . . . The measurement of blood pressure, while subject to standardized criteria, has been standardized separately for each nation and even the technical prerequisites of measurement vary.
—Dr. Manfred Pflanz

- An American opera singer in Vienna consulted an Austrian doctor, who prescribed suppositories for her headache. Not used to receiving headache medication in this form, she ate one.
- A British general practitioner took his wife to a North Carolina clinic where he was temporarily working to show her the position American women customarily assume for a pelvic examination. Her judgment: "Why, that's barbaric!" Her husband performed the examination with women lying on their sides and, while he was ridiculed by the other North Carolina doctors, he soon found he had a queue of women outside his office who had heard he examined "the English way."
- A French professor on sabbatical in California suffered an attack of angina pectoris, for which his doctors recommended

immediate coronary bypass surgery. The professor consented, not realizing that at the time American rates of frequency for coronary bypass were twenty-eight times that of some European countries and that later studies were to show that bypasses rarely have to be done immediately, if at all.

• A young American working in Germany was told by her German gynecologist to take mud baths rather than antibiotics to treat her vaginal infection. "I don't want to sit in mud," wailed the woman later to a colleague. "All I want is a couple of pills!"

World travelers who have had to see a doctor in a foreign country have usually discovered that medicine is not quite the international science that the medical profession would like us to believe. Not only do ways of delivering medical care differ from country to country; so does the medicine that is delivered. The differences are so great that one country's treatment of choice may be considered malpractice across the border.

Some of the most commonly prescribed drugs in France, drugs to dilate the cerebral blood vessels, are considered ineffective in England and America; an obligatory immunization against tuberculosis in France, BCG, is almost impossible to obtain in the United States. German doctors prescribe from six to seven times the amount of digitalislike drugs as their colleagues in France and England, but they prescribe fewer antibiotics, with some German doctors maintaining antibiotics shouldn't be used unless the patient is sick enough to be in the hospital. Doses of the same drug may vary drastically, with some nationalities getting ten to twenty times what other nationals get. French people have seven times the chance of getting drugs in suppository form as do Americans. In the late 1960s American surgery rates were twice those of England; and the intervening years have seen this surgery gap widen, not close. Rates for individual operations vary even more. One study found three times as many mastectomies in New England as in England or Sweden, even though the rate of breast cancer was similar;

another found that German-speaking countries had three times the rate of appendectomies of other countries; there are six times the number of coronary bypasses per capita in America when compared to England. Even if the operation has the same general name it may be done differently: West German doctors perform mostly vaginal hysterectomies; French doctors commonly perform subtotal hysterectomies; and English and U.S. doctors favor total abdominal hysterectomies.

The same clinical signs may even receive different diagnoses. Often, all one must do to acquire a disease is to enter a country where that disease is recognized—leaving the country will either cure the malady or turn it into something else. The American schizophrenic of a few years ago might well have found his disease called manic-depressive disease or even neurosis had he sought a second opinion in Britain; in France he likely would have been diagnosed as having a delusional psychosis. The Frenchman suffering from spasmophilia or the German from vasovegetative dystonia would be considered merely neurotic in Britain or perhaps a victim of panic disorder in the United States if he were considered sick at all.

Blood pressure considered treatably high in the United States might be considered normal in England; and the low blood pressure treated with eighty-five drugs as well as hydrotherapy and spa treatments in Germany would entitle its sufferer to lower life insurance rates in the United States.

The differences are most marked for minor complaints but not at all limited to them. "Plenty of people," wrote Dr. M. N. G. Dukes in the *British Medical Journal,* "are still dying of diseases which other people do not believe in." One World Health Organization study found that doctors from different countries diagnosed different causes of death even when shown identical information from the same death certificates. There was a considerable amount of disagreement in coding infective and parasitic disease, "other heart" diseases, hypertension, pneumonia, nephritis and nephrosis, and diseases of the newborn. "There was fairly good agreement . . . on whether a death was due to a malignant neoplasm [cancer] or not, but less agreement on the location of neoplasms . . . ," a finding confirmed by another study sponsored by the American National Cancer Institute.

A psychiatric assessment of which patients are dangerous can result in their being locked up; yet when psychiatrists from six countries tried to agree on who was dangerous, the overall level of agreement was under 50 percent for three-quarters of the cases considered, and the psychiatrists did not agree any more among themselves than did nonpsychiatrists.

Even within a given country, of course, not all doctors diagnose and treat identically, and the differences among different specialists can often be particularly marked. But many comparisons have shown that while doctors within a given country differ somewhat, doctors from different countries differ even more.

How can medicine, which is commonly supposed to be a science, particularly in the United States, be so different in four countries whose peoples are so similar genetically? The answer is that while medicine benefits from a certain amount of scientific input, culture intervenes at every step of the way.

Take, for example, a very common situation in medicine. A patient is excessively tired, and makes an appointment with his doctor.

Already, a difference emerges. In England the patient would be obliged by the National Health Service to make an appointment with his general practitioner, whereas in tne United States there are so few general practitioners that the patient would commonly choose some sort of specialist such as a gynecologist, pediatrician, or internist. Since even within a country different types of doctors treat the same illness differently, the different ratios of specialists will already have wide repercussions.

The physician faced with a tired patient will have several choices, since fatigue can be a sign of a number of diseases, including viral illness, depression, cancer, and heart disease. The doctor can examine the patient, and the frequency and thoroughness of examinations differ markedly from country to country. He can order tests, and here, too, enormous differences have been documented. He can delay, telling the patient to wait and see if his energy returns. Or he can come up with a diagnosis that will reassure the patient and hope that the placebo effect will then cure whatever it is. Often the physician feels this last approach is the best thing he can do for his patient.

The diagnosis he reaches in such a case will be strongly influenced by culture: what he learned in medical school, what he knows other doctors say, and what he knows will reassure the patient. A liver crisis will reassure a French patient while it would alarm an American one; the diagnosis of "a virus" would probably have opposite effects on each.

Many of the more scientifically minded physicians in all countries discount such "wastebasket diagnoses," claiming that they are really not scientific medicine at all. "In France, we would call vague digestive troubles a liver crisis; in the United States you would call it a food allergy. You prescribe anything at all, because it's not a scientific diagnosis, but rather a different use of placebos," said Dr. Henri Pequignot, a professor of medicine at Paris's Hôpital Cochin.

Most patients and most doctors, however, don't realize that they are using placebos, and, as we shall see later, such wastebasket diagnoses influence so-called scientific medicine in a number of ways.

But for the time being let us accept Dr. Pequignot's comment that such diagnoses and treatments are unimportant, and look instead at what he would admit is "scientific medicine." Suppose, for example, that a doctor in one country decides to perform a scientific study. In planning his study, the doctor or other medical scientist must decide whether it will be a randomized, controlled trial (RCT), in which patients are divided into at least two groups, the two groups treated differently, and the results eventually compared. The strength of such trials is that they are usually considered to provide the most scientific answer; the problem is that patients must be treated differently and the results then compared, and many doctors find this ethically distasteful. RCTs are also difficult to organize and carry out. While RCTs have to some extent been adopted in all the countries, they are done most often in England. One of their most vocal advocates, Dr. Archibald Cochrane, wrote in his book *Effectiveness and Efficiency*: "If some such index as the number of RCTs per 1,000 doctors per year for all countries were worked out and a map of the world shaded according to the level of the index (black being the highest), one would see the UK in black and scattered black patches in Scandinavia, the USA and a few other countries: The rest would be nearly white."

In the chapters that follow, the reason RCTs are considered so differently, as well as why it is easier to have a placebo-controlled trial in England than in America, will be considered. But for the moment, let us simply consider this point: *If a study is not performed as an RCT, it will probably not be accepted for publication in the English medical literature.* Which brings us to our next point: *Doctors in one country rarely read the medical literature of any country but their own.*

Dr. A. M. W. Porter, a general practitioner in Surrey, England, interviewed French and British doctors and found that the British doctors couldn't name a single French medical journal, and the French were only able to name an average of slightly over one British journal, mostly *The Lancet.* My own observations would suggest that the French are even more ignorant of the German medical literature, and vice versa. Communication may be somewhat better between the British and the Americans. But when a vice president of the American Cancer Society was informed in the mid-1970s of a study published in the *British Medical Journal* that showed women treated for early breast cancer by "tylectomy" (the British author's term for lumpectomy) survived just as long as those treated by radical mastectomy, his reply was: "We don't read much foreign literature here."

As a result of this mutual ignorance, the English and Americans are constantly rediscovering what the French and Germans have known for a long time, and vice versa. Dr. Marcel-Francis Kahn, a professor of rheumatology at Hôpital Bichat in Paris, pointed out that while a letter in the 1981 volume of the journal *Arthritis and Rheumatism* credited Churchill and his associates as the first to document disc-space infections in bacterial endocarditis, there had already been no fewer than ten articles in the French literature devoted to the subject, the first published in 1965.

Doctors claim that they stay on top of other countries' medical advances by attending international meetings, but presenting a paper at an international meeting is no guarantee that anyone is listening. To start with, there's the problem of language. Even the best simultaneous interpreter is going to have trouble dealing with the fact that *peptic ulcer* and *bronchitis* don't mean the same things in Britain that they do in the United States; that the U.S. *appendectomy* becomes the British *appendicectomy;* that the French tendency to exaggerate means there are never headaches in France, only migraines, and that the French often refer to real migraines as "liver crises"; that the German language has no word for chest pain, forcing the German patient to talk of heart pain, and that when a German doctor says "cardiac insufficiency" he may simply mean that the patient is tired.

A similar situation prevails in psychiatric language. "Even though bilingual dictionaries may give the impression that the English adjectives paranoid, paranoiac and delusional are the exact equivalents of French *paranoïde, paranoïaque* and *délirant,* French- and English-speaking psychiatrists use these terms quite differently and with vastly divergent frequencies," wrote Dr. Pierre Pichot, a French psychiatrist who is past president of the International Psychiatric Association.

Then, too, not all interpreters are top-notch, and the headphones may not work; at best they are irritating. At small meetings where scientists discuss a highly specialized topic in one language, communication is likely to be good; at large international congresses, doctors usually go to the sessions where their countrymen are speaking and spend the rest of the time sightseeing.

Dr. Sakari Härö, chief of the Department of Planning and Evaluation of the National Board of Health in Helsinki, Finland, put it this way: "At a meeting, the Finns tend to group with the English. The Germans stay together as a bloc, as do the Southern and Eastern Europeans. At a meeting I seldom discuss with the French—I'm half sleeping when French is being spoken."

If the language barrier is breached, and people understand the words, they will probably start to criticize the science. If a French or German doctor gives a paper, for example, a British doctor will often get up in the question-and-answer period and say scathingly, "I think it is scandalous that we are still hearing about uncontrolled trials."

Even if the science is understood and accepted, there may be no agreement as to what the study means for the practice of medicine. This is true even within a country: studies may show the consequence of a certain course of action, i.e., a treatment, but judging whether the consequence is good or bad can be highly subjective. Dr. E. M. Glaser, for example, writing in the *British Medical Journal*, pointed out the wide disparity of conclusions that had been drawn in the same issue of the *BMJ*. One paper, reporting a near death from eating licorice, had no comment on future safety; another, on intestinal bypass operations for obesity, reported statistically significant liver damage in all patients studied and a 4 percent mortality but concluded that "further careful evaluation of the effects of intestinal bypass operations is required"; and a third that showed an adverse reaction in one of 1,000 persons given an intravenous anesthetic induction agent concluded that this rate of side effects made the intravenous injection unacceptable.

If such very subjective conclusions concerning future courses of action can be drawn in a single issue of one medical journal, the possible range of subjectivity from country to country is, of course, even greater. Consider, for example, a study that shows that giving chemotherapy to elderly patients with cancer prolongs their lives by an average of a few months but also causes them severe, intractable, drug-induced vomiting. If one believes that length of life is the most important criterion, this study would indicate that such patients should be given chemotherapy; if one believes quality of life is more important it might indicate that chemotherapy should not be given.

In fact, the American authors of this particular paper felt the added months justified a recommendation for chemotherapy; Englishmen who commented on it in the *BMJ* felt this recommendation was off base. In neither commentary did the authors recommend that patients be asked how they felt about the matter.

If a study fits into the general scheme of medical thinking in a country, it is likely to be widely cited. This is particularly true if it shows that a drug is effective or an operation works, because the drug company and the surgeons concerned will see that the study gets written and talked about. If the study goes against medical thinking, medical professionals find it quite easy to ignore one study amid the thousands that are published each month. An RCT performed in 1922, for example, showed that women whose pubic hair was shaved before giving birth had more infections than those whose pubic hair wasn't shaved, and these results were shown again in 1965. Yet many hospital services in England and America (not in France) continued the practice, probably due to some puritanical feeling that pubic hair *should* be shaved. A 1986 paper in a prominent German medical journal proved that the horse-chestnut extracts already widely used in Germany to treat problems of the circulation actually do work—and I'll wager that while the study will be widely cited in Germany, it will be completely ignored in the United States.

The Common Market countries theoretically allow free movement of goods and services among them. But the fact that one country allows a drug to be put on its market does not automatically put the drug on the market in other countries. In fact, in no case since the establishment of the Common Market have all the members accepted a drug just because it was accepted in one country. According to Dr. Gerald Jones of the Department of Health and Social Security in the United Kingdom, the differences were always related to risk-benefit ratios of the drugs: "We all use the same guidelines, yet different opinions are reached on the same preclinical or clinical data."

In general, doctors in all countries—except, as we shall see, England—favor studies that suggest new types of treatments rather than studies that show current treatments are unnecessary. For example, Dr. Umberto Veronesi, director of the Italian National Cancer Institute in Milan, observed, "We did a trial showing that in malignant melanoma, after removal of the primary tumor, there is no need to remove the regional lymph nodes if they are not palpably involved. We followed up 600 patients for 12 years, and our results, published five years ago, are very clear. But the reaction of general surgeons has been strong and hostile—the majority of them still remove the regional lymph nodes."

In the United States, coronary artery bypass surgery was widely adopted before any studies had shown it to be effective in preventing death or disability; yet, on the other hand, the practice of allowing women who have had a cesarean section to deliver vaginally a subsequent time will probably not be adopted—despite some twenty studies showing that under proper conditions such a practice is safe. The popularity of coronary bypass surgery concords with the American culture biases of aggressive treatment and with the American view of the body as a machine; while reducing the number of cesarean sections would contradict American values in favoring nonintervention and being mainly of psychological value to delivering women.

It is, of course, easier for doctors to reject a foreign study. Dr. Fritz Beller, a professor of gynecology at the University of Münster in West Germany, refers to the phenomenon as Beller's Rule Number One: A method developed on one continent has difficulty being accepted on another. One unnamed American researcher noted that, for many of his colleagues, "If we don't describe it first, our first reaction is always negative. We are very chauvinistic and have the attitude that if we haven't found something, it's probably wrong."

Rejection of study results may also be based on how doctors feel their patients would react. In response to evidence that cholera vaccination was of little value, the health authorities of one unnamed developed country explained: "The fear of cholera is strongly felt by a large part of the population which still trusts vaccination practice as a control measure against the disease. We feel that our population, as well as that of other countries, would not agree to drop a protective measure, even if it has been scientifically demonstrated to be of little value."

The way the doctor is paid, and the organization of medical care, will also influence acceptance. Dr. Henk Lamberts, a Dutch GP active in international organizations, said, "When you see a patient whose wound has been treated by a Spanish doctor, it will have two sutures, since in Spain doctors are paid by treating the wound. An Austrian doctor would have put in six sutures, and the Belgian doctor would have put in as many sutures as he could, as they are paid by the number of sutures."

Dr. Lamberts emphasized that he didn't mean to sound cynical. "Belgian culture values sutures, so they are put in. It's appreciated, so he gets paid for it."

The widespread ignorance that medicine in highly developed countries can be so different has a number of serious implications. First, all sorts of unjustified conclusions are currently being drawn from international statistics. A press handout concerning rates of coronary artery disease in various countries, for example, showed the rate to be low in West Germany. While the person who compiled the release had copied the figures correctly from international statistics, he was unaware that while West Germany reports relatively low rates of coronary artery disease, the country reports much higher rates of "other" heart disease than do England and the United States. If the rates of coronary artery disease and other heart disease are taken together, as it has been suggested they should, West Germany, England, and the United States have similar rates of heart disease.

Second, the different ways that different countries treat the same disease constitute a sort of natural experiment; yet because most people are unaware of the experiment in the first place, they are unable to draw the conclusions that might result. For example, French doctors have widely prescribed calcium for a number of years, and a closer examination of osteoporosis rates there might help illuminate the role of calcium in this disease. As a corollary, a greater understanding of medical culture bias might predict the country in which side effects will first surface—or will be hidden. The neural side effects of bismuth were first discovered in France, where very high doses were prescribed for constipation; conversely, the very serious side effects that an antihypertensive drug, Selacryn, had on the liver were underestimated in France, perhaps because the French, who frequently attribute liver troubles to rich food and drink or a constitutionally "fragile" liver, would be less likely to see a drug as the culprit.

Finally, many of the medical mistakes made in each country can be best understood by cultural biases that blind both the medical profession and patients, causing them to accept some treatments too quickly and other treatments reluctantly or not at all. Understanding the cultural basis for these mistakes can perhaps prevent them—or at least lessen their impact.

France:

Cartesian Thinking and the Terrain

In France we may not have oil, but we have ideas.
—French government propaganda
widely broadcast in the 1970s

There's no money, we have no great laboratories. The only things
that we can have are ideas and patients and this disease.
—French AIDS researcher
Dr. Jean Marie Andrieu

I don't act. I am. I operate without sterilized gloves. I trust germs.
They devour me, they ravage me. It's violent.
—French actor Gérard Depardieu

My first initiation into the very large role cultural values play
in medicine came in the summer of 1972, about a year after I
had arrived in France, when I covered a meeting on nonmu-
tilating treatments for breast cancer in Strasbourg, France.

The meeting got off to a roaring start with its organizer,
Professor Charles Gros, giving a slide show on the breast and
breast cancer in the history of art, referring to the breast as
"man's pleasure" and "woman's narcissism." The exhibitors
seemed to enjoy the theme—there were breasts everywhere
in the exhibition area, including one entire wall of plastic
breasts so pointed it seemed that anyone who accidentally pushed
against it would suffer major puncture wounds. By the third
day everyone was booing slides that showed a bad cosmetic

result, which seemed as appropriate a response as any in that setting.

My initial response was shock. Like many American women I had been raised on magazine articles declaring: "I gave up my breast to save my life." I had assumed that the trade-off was a necessary one, the choice black and white—that no serious person would consider a woman's breast more important than her life.

Except, as I learned during those days in Strasbourg, the issues weren't black and white. Studies had already shown that breast-saving operations, at least in certain cases, gave as good a chance of survival as the radical mastectomy. Moreover, at least some of the studies showing this dated back to the 1930s, when a Finnish radiotherapist and a British surgeon were already getting good results treating breast cancer without removing the breast. These good results were susceptible to criticisms of "selection bias," i.e., that women with small cancers were selected for the less radical treatments and that such women were known to have a good survival whatever the treatment. On the basis of these early results there was no way to tell whether they would have had a *better* survival with the radical mastectomy. But recently an English surgeon, John Hayward, had shown that women with small tumors treated by lumpectomy plus radiotherapy survived just as long as women treated by radical mastectomy. The only question remaining was whether this good result seen after ten years of treatment would continue over many years. And Mr. Hayward (British surgeons are known as Mister, not Doctor, in a sort of reverse snobbism dating from the days of the barber-surgeons, when surgeons were not *allowed* to call themselves doctors) pointed out that even if the radical mastectomy proved to give a better survival, the difference would be small, with only 5 to 10 percent of women benefiting from it.

In the light of this evidence, the French point of view—that one should enjoy breasts, even at a breast cancer meeting—became more understandable. Facing certain death rather than lose a breast might not make a lot of sense, but facing a slightly decreased statistical chance of being alive in twenty years seemed a reasonable trade-off. Thinking about the meeting afterward, I was glad the French were emphasizing the importance of aesthetic, sexual, and psychological concerns.

But the meeting was an interesting exercise not only in how values differ, but also in how thought, including medical thought, itself differs. The French were ready to accept the English trial as well as other, uncontrolled, trials as definitive. The English thought there should be more trials, and kept trying to point out to the French participants why. And the Americans mostly didn't come.

To understand French medical thinking, one must first understand that the French, more than just about any other nationality, value thinking as an activity in itself. Americans value doers, the French value thinkers. While intellectuals may make the obituary column in the United States, French intellectuals regularly make the front page, sometimes even when they are admitted to the hospital, which French people are likely to consider is due to their overwork from thinking. Professor Marcel-Francis Kahn of Hôpital Bichat in Paris explained that French people grew up reading biographies of famous artists and writers that ended: "Epuisé par le travail, il est mort" (exhausted by work, he died), thoroughly ingraining the notion that intellectual work is even more exhausting than physical labor.

The late Spanish diplomat Salvador de Madariaga defined the Englishman as the man of action, the Spaniard as the man of passion, and the Frenchman as the man of thought. "The Englishman, when thinking, meditates on action," he wrote. "The Frenchman, when acting, executes his thoughts." What the Frenchman wants from action, according to de Madariaga, is that action should obey the laws of reason, that it should fall into a clear order of things. Unlike English law, which grows out of past cases, French law under Napoleon was written into a code, still in use today, that tries to anticipate and regulate the social order. Even the casual visitor to France can see signs of this in the Paris *métro*, where the priorities of seating are listed in great detail. Unlike English measurements, a sloppy mishmash that grew out of tradition, French metric measurements are totally logical. Unlike English and American ways of paying the doctor for services, which in their very different ways pay for costs after they are incurred, the French system has established, in advance, exactly how much money the doctor or patient will be reimbursed for each drug and each procedure performed. Given the value the French place on thinking, it is not surprising that consultations (without any associated acts) are better reimbursed in France than they are in Germany and that the average length of a doctor visit in France is much longer than in Germany.

As a consequence of prices being fixed in advance, the only way the French doctor can increase his income is by performing more services. "If an American doctor wants to double his income, he doubles his fees; if a French doctor wants to double his income, he takes out twice as many appendixes," recounted one French doctor.

The French way of thinking is often referred to, with admiration within France and pejoratively outside of France, as Cartesian, after the French philosopher Descartes. Descartes's love of logic and theory and his disdain for practical data greatly influenced French thought. Descartes tried to clear his mind of all preconceived notions and then started with the famous *Cogito ergo sum* (I think, therefore I am). From there, he proceeded logically to "prove" the universe.

"The quest for the touchstones and talismans of the French conscience still leads unerringly to Descartes," wrote Sanche de Gramont in his book *The French.* "Descartes embarked on the highest adventure of the mind: to conquer the universe without ever leaving his study," according to de Gramont, an offspring of French nobility who moved to America and eventually changed his name to Ted Morgan. "It does not matter that his findings were inaccurate, as long as the method was convincing. . . . A general who devises a perfect battle plan with incomplete information about enemy capacity, and goes on to elegant defeat, is Cartesian. An engineer from the ministry of Ponts et Chaussées who designs a bridge for a town on the Drôme which he has never visited, on the basis of topographical maps, is Cartesian. When he is told that the bridge has been washed away by floods he merely says: 'That is impossible.' "

The astronomer Urbain-Jean Leverrier, according to de Gramont, discovered the planet Neptune on the basis of calculations, and when the planet was first seen he refused to look at it. Louis Pasteur, who did perform experiments, commented on a treatise on fermentation by the physiologist Claude Bernard: "All this is wrong, and to prove it I will conduct an experiment the outcome of which I can predict beforehand."

More recently the late Jacques Monod, the Nobel Prize–winning molecular biologist who became head of the Pasteur Institute, said: "I have sometimes used the trick of writing the paper before the experiments were done—not publishing it, of course—but the discipline is very good for choosing which experiments should be done."

I was interviewing Monod about the Pasteur Institute flu vaccine, which had been launched with great fanfare in France ("Victory Over the Flu" was the headline in *Le Monde*). English and American flu experts remained extremely skeptical about the vaccine, mainly because it had been announced effective on the basis of theory and not because it had been shown to prevent flu. When I relayed these criticisms to Professor Monod, he was quick to point out that these were not criticisms of theory or results but of principle. Clinical trials, he said, were not easy to do in France because of the philosophy of the medical profession. "I am very confident about vaccinating large numbers of people without challenge experiments," he said.

More recently, French AIDS researchers held a press conference to announce their "results" with cyclosporine. In fact, these results comprised treatment of six patients, on only two of whom preliminary lab findings were available, and they had been using the drug for only about a week. American researchers denounced the results as the "crummiest type of anecdotal evidence." What they did not understand, of course, was that it was not the evidence that was of importance in France but the idea—an intellectually elegant approach to treating AIDS.

When Professor W. W. Holland, professor of clinical epidemiology and social medicine at St. Thomas's Hospital Medical School in London, visited France, he found a Cartesian attitude even toward such a mundane task as evaluating results of health care. "Little of the research work commissioned appears to be concerned with outcome," he wrote; "most is concerned with process. Perhaps the best example of this is multiphasic screening, which has been running for five years in France. It is supposed to have undergone proper evaluation, but no paper has been published and the methodology and techniques are such that it is unlikely that any clear conclusion about its value will ever be reached." One World Health Organization epidemiologist referred to epidemiology in France as *l'art pour l'art*. In actual clinical practice, Cartesianism often means, according to Dr. Henk Lamberts, a Dutch general practitioner, "if the idea is good, the body has to follow."

When French women started to complain that their supposedly "painless childbirth," as the Lamaze method is referred to in France, had actually been for some of them unbearably painful, one French obstetrician wrote in *Le Monde* that it was *impossible* that a woman well prepared in the Lamaze technique could suffer pain and that no painkillers or anesthesia were needed. If a woman did suffer, he said, it was because she had started her training too late or had not worked at it hard enough, or that the obstetrical team had not taken the method seriously.

Doctors from other countries working in international groups often comment on how difficult the French are to work with; a lot of the difficulty seems to be due to the Cartesian ways the French view problems. The English Dr. Alastair Mason, for example, said of the French he worked with on a committee on biomedical information: "Their thought processes are so different from mine. They have huge grandiose schemes and I try to come up with little, practical ones."

Dr. Lamberts, who worked on a classification system with the French, claimed that they will insist, for example, that high blood pressure always has an effect on the target organ and that that must be in the classification. "We ask, What are the figures? and they have none. If you have no hard facts, we say, we won't accept your classification."

Some of the drugs popular in France and not elsewhere fall into the category of good ideas that lack good data to support their efficacy. One of the most common classes of drug prescribed in France is the "supposed" vasodilators, drugs supposed to dilate the blood vessels in the brains of older persons suffering from the effects of senility. In a study by the Office of Health Economics in London, this was the third most commonly prescribed class of drugs in France in 1982. According to Dr. Henri Pequignot, of Hôpital Cochin in Paris, the idea that such drugs might work was originally English, although since there is no evidence that they do work, these types of peripheral vasodilators are not widely used in England or America.

I asked Dr. René Royer, a doctor and pharmacologist who works with the French department of health, in the fall of 1985 if the government had any plans to ban these drugs, considering the lack of proof of their efficacy. "No," he said. "We're not certain that they *don't* work."

Another very common practice is the almost systematic prescription of lactobacillus every time an antibiotic is prescribed, supposedly to prevent the stomach upsets that antibiotics can cause. This practice had its origin with Ilya Metchnikoff, the Russian scientist who lived in France and received a Nobel Prize. Metchnikoff, who lived in the preantibiotic era, believed that the secret of eternal youth could be found in Bulgarian yogurt, of which he kept a large pot in the laboratory; visitors were often invited to have some. When antibiotics were discovered, it was shown that they change the bacterial composition of the intestinal tract; and the idea arose of replacing the "good" bacteria destroyed by the drugs with lactobacillus, which already had a very positive image because of Metchnikoff.

The idea was good, but it's never been shown that the "good" bacteria can in fact be replaced in the intestine any faster with lactobacillus than without it. In addition, since lactobacillus is found in both yogurt and cheese, which the French eat a lot of, they probably would need less lactobacillus than other nationalities even if it were effective. Why, then, does the practice of prescribing lactobacillus and yogurt continue? In the opinion of Dr. Jacques Acar, a professor in infectious diseases, it "proves that the doctor is doing something for the patient. When a French doctor writes a prescription, there's always a part that is aimed at raising the morale." (The French may be vindicated for having done the right thing for the wrong reason. In the summer of 1984, American researchers showed that lactobacillus seems to metabolize cholesterol; and the French practice of eating so much yogurt and lactobacillus may play a role in their low rate of heart attacks. Perhaps Metchnikoff was right.)

Another French practice, taking the temperature rectally rather than orally, derives from a good idea that nevertheless inconveniences the patient and can have negative side effects. Rectal temperatures are more accurate than oral temperatures, but most English and Americans would say that in most cases such a degree of accuracy is unnecessary and not worth the inconvenience. But the French almost always take their temperatures this way, and oral thermometers, at least a few years ago, were not to be found in French pharmacies. "I personally don't trust oral temperatures," said one French-educated pediatrician now living in New York, who attributed the American practice of oral temperatures to puritanism. "What if the patient has just eaten ice cream?"

In fact, the French practice causes rather significant side effects: the director of an emergency hemorrhoid service in Paris said that "thermometer ulcers" are a common cause of rectal bleeding in France. "Not only do the French take their temperatures rectally, but many of the thermometers are pointed," he said. The practice will continue, according to one Frenchman, because: "Who would put a thermometer in his mouth that might have been in someone else's rectum? Nobody, which is why we'll probably never switch over in France."

Cartesian thinking can explain many of the ways French psychiatry differs from that in other Western European countries. While most countries accepted some form of the classification system worked out by the German Emil Kraepelin, France never did, objecting to Kraepelin's empiricism, which, as Pierre Pichot describes, "allowed him to be content with arguments based on development, and on his lack of theoretical concepts, which had the result that his classification, 'far from being systematic, [is] rather a nomenclature.' " To this day the classification of psychiatric disease in France is quite different from that in Germany, England, and the United States.

Through the mid-1960s French psychiatrists described emotional disturbances as disturbances of the intellect and encouraged their rational control in terms that suggested a moral imperative, according to Sherry Turkle in her book *Psychoanalytic Politics*. Turkle points out that Cartesian thinking and the value placed on intellect also help explain the very different path psychoanalysis took in France: "The psychiatric resistance to psychoanalysis allowed it a long period of incubation in the world of artists and writers before a significant breakthrough into medicine, a pattern which reinforced the French tendency to take ideas and invest them with philosophical and ideological significance instead of turning them outward toward problem-solving."

When the "French Freud," in the person of Jacques Lacan, finally arrived, wrote Turkle, he treated psychoanalysis less as a way to adjustment or problem solving than as an intellectual exercise. "One would not expect the national versions of psychoanalysis to be any less varied than the national versions of Calvinism," wrote Turkle. "An American patient, nursed on the

Horatio Alger story and on dramatic tales of biological or spiritual ancestors battling it out at the frontier, can respond to a picture of his psyche which emphasizes the struggles of the ego with the demands of a difficult reality. A French patient who has been doing *explication du texte* and memorizing literary aphorisms since grade school might be more receptive to a psychoanalysis which presents itself as a form of textual analysis of the unconscious."

According to Lacan, a critical point in the development of a child is seeing himself in a mirror for the first time, adding a sort of visual dimension to Descartes's *Cogito ergo sum*, making it, "I see myself, therefore I am."

This visual, intuitive aspect of French thought has numerous consequences, particularly in diagnosis. English thought works by enumeration or inventory, and Dr. Françoise Rothman, who studied medicine in both the United States and France, says that in the United States she learned to make diagnoses by considering all the possible diagnoses and eliminating them one by one. In France, by contrast, she learned to make diagnoses by putting all the symptoms together, like pieces in a puzzle.

"French thought does not take, it sees. It sees all there is to be seen and everything in its place," wrote de Madariaga. While American companies make job applicants take multiple-choice tests, French companies are more likely to have them submit a sample of their handwriting to be analyzed. A type of article that in English might be described as an "anatomy" in France is described as a *"radioscopie"* (X ray).

As a consequence, while the American doctor will rely more heavily on laboratory tests, in France doctors seem to have a greater tendency to diagnose after a look at the patient or the X ray.

Dr. Ralph L. Thompson, in his *Glimpses of Medical Europe*, published in 1908, recounts a visit to the dermatology clinic at the Hôpital St. Louis in Paris: "I went there primarily to see the much-talked-of 'bald-headed clinic' of Sabouraud. Everybody has heard of this clinic, where those who have lost their hair come by hundreds, and of the great Sabouraud who pulls a hair (provided there is one remaining) from your head, glances at it, and says, 'Yes, I can cure you; go into the next room'; to another, 'You may be benefitted, wait here'; and to a third, 'Go and buy a wig; nothing can be done for you.' It is said that Sabouraud can tell your moral character, the amount of your yearly income, and what you have eaten for breakfast, by looking at a root of one of your hairs."

More recently, an American asked her highly recommended French doctor if eating half a grapefruit a day would be a good way to get her vitamin C. The doctor said it would, provided that the grapefruit was from Florida, not Israel. "I can tell by looking at you that you are very acidic," the doctor said, "and Israeli grapefruit would make you even more so."

The French do "look well," in the opinion of several observers, including Professor Hans Schadewaldt of the Institute of the History of Medicine in Düsseldorf, who was a prisoner of war in France. Perhaps this is why when French, English, and German psychiatrists were shown the same patient, French doctors saw an average of 10 symptoms per patient, compared to 8.4 for the English and 7.5 for the Germans. French psychiatrists were particularly likely to perceive symptoms like retardation, perplexity, lack of energy, and paranoid ideas.

Radiologists in all countries must by the very nature of their work make intuitive, visual diagnoses, and perhaps because of their tendency to favor such thinking anyway, the French seem to give a high prestige to radiologists and to radiology. While there are twice as many anesthesiologists in England as in France, there are more radiologists in France than in England. And the number of radiologists doesn't tell the whole story. Dr. Kahn explains that other specialists in France receive much more training in interpreting X rays than those in the United States and England, where most interpretation is left to the radiologist. In his own specialty, rheumatology, for example, there are courses and tests in radiorheumatology as well as books devoted to the subject. "I'm certain that French doctors on the whole use many more X rays than American doctors," he says.

One type of radiologic exam, the hysterosalpingogram, or radiology of the uterus and fallopian tubes, is performed in France for conditions that would be diagnosed with a dilatation and curetage in West Germany, England, and the United States. Hysterosalpingograms are performed in these countries, but almost exclusively for the investigation of infertility. In a recent French text of hysterosalpingography, the stated indications for the procedure include fibroid tumors, endometrial hyperplasia, endometriosis, placement of IUDs, scars from cesarean section, and normal and pathologic pregnancies.

Several French doctors said they couldn't imagine performing a D&C without having first performed a hysterosalpingogram, a situation that is decidedly not the case in England, West Germany, and America, where the procedure is considered to give much too high a dose of radiation for such routine use. "They are very keen on radiology here," said Mr. Stanley Bond, a British gynecologic surgeon who moved his practice to France. "They do hysterosalpingograms for all sorts of purposes we would never dream of using them for."

A German gynecologist, Dr. Fritz Beller, refused to believe me when I told him that French doctors used hysterosalpingograms for such a wide range of diagnoses. "Hysterosalpingography is not diagnostic for ovarian cysts and fibroid tumors," he said. "We only do them [hysterosalpingograms] for sterility, and we're going to laparoscopy for that!"

Professor Maurice Laval-Jeantet, whom I interviewed in October 1985, noted that ultrasound was now used for many of the same conditions that used to be diagnosed with hysterosalpingography. But, he said, French doctors still liked to do a hysterosalpingogram after the ultrasound. "Many gynecologists prefer the hysterosalpingogram to the sonogram," he said, "or they'll use the sonogram for screening and then do a hysterosalpingogram for diagnosis. The sonogram doesn't give as good an image as the hysterosalpingogram—and the French love *la belle image.*"

Dr. A. Netter, a retired French professor of medical gynecology, thought the differing use of the two diagnostic procedures was largely a question of tradition. The hysterosalpingogram, he said, was originally developed by a French gynecologist, Dr. Claude Béclère, who was the son of a radiologist. But Dr. Netter suggested two other reasons the tradition might have "taken" in France and not in England or America. While gynecologists in most countries are surgeons, in France specialists known as medical gynecologists typically handle routine problems. "For a nonsurgeon, a hysterosalpingogram is much easier to perform than a D & C." He also suggested that a D & C, which tends to give a diagnosis of cancer or not cancer, fits in with the black-and-white view of medicine prevalent in the United States, whereas hysterosalpingograms fit in with the more nuanced view prevailing in France.

But a number of French doctors cited a different reason for their reluctance to use D & C's for diagnostic purposes: synechia, or intrauterine adhesions, may be formed as a side effect of D & C's. Such adhesions can cause infertility problems, they say, and therefore a D & C should not be used in young women.

"Synechia!" exclaimed the German Dr. Beller. "I've only seen about three cases of synechia in my life," a sentiment echoed by other non-French doctors.

But the French may have the last word. Dr. Beller was interviewed in 1979, and since then at least one study of infertile women showed that many had intrauterine adhesions, and that nearly all of these women had previously had a D & C, either for abortion or as a diagnostic procedure.

French fairy tales don't simply end with "And they lived happily ever after," but add, "and had lots of children." France has been concerned about its low birth rate for years and worries that in a few generations there will be no more French men and women. The French birth rate is currently below the replacement level, at 1.94 children per woman in 1982, but it is higher than the birth rate in West Germany, 1.42 children per woman, and in Britain, 1.81 children per woman. Perhaps the incentives given to pregnant women and young families—totally free medical care plus *allocations familiales*, periodic payments for each child regardless of income—have had their effect.

The concern about fertility is reflected in a number of French medical practices. The French made a concerted effort to reduce their infant mortality rate and did so within a few years, making it lower than that in England, West Germany, and the United States. It was French researchers who recently published a study on the subject of why older women have trouble conceiving. "Why this should be seems to have intrigued French researchers in particular," commented a *Lancet* editorial. Similarly, while Americans tend to emphasize that the risks of the various methods of birth control are not as high as "the overwhelming risk of pregnancy," the French are more likely to emphasize the risks of birth control.

Although French law does not expressly forbid sterilization, well-publicized criminal prosecutions in 1937 for sterilizations made French doctors aware that they could be prosecuted for "mutilation," a fear not assuaged by the continuing opposition to sterilization of the Ordre des Médecins, a group to which all French doctors must belong. As a consequence, at least until very recently, doctors would perform sterilizations only if for compelling reasons. "It's not because it's illegal that we don't do it," said Dr. Alain Fournié, an obstetrician-gynecologist from Toulouse. "We do occasionally perform sterilizations—but exceptionally before the age of thirty-five and rarely before forty, and only after a talk with the woman, her husband, and the opinion of a psychiatrist." A French medical journal article discussing contraception in the diabetic patient said that before tubal ligation was considered, the patient should have severe degenerative complications, kidney failure, high blood pressure, proliferative retinopathy of the eye, at least two living children, be over thirty-five, psychologically stable, and in agreement with the partner that tubal ligation was the answer.

Prior to getting a prescription for contraceptive pills, a French woman is usually sent for cholesterol, triglyceride, and blood sugar tests, measurements not commonly taken in the United States before a birth-control pill is prescribed. According to Dr. Netter, this practice dates to one French doctor, Jean-Luc De Gennes, an endocrinologist who found that women with abnormal lipid metabolism who took the pill developed many medical problems. In Dr. Netter's opinion, "It's not certain that the practice of doing lipid studies on all women who want to take the pill is justified. Doctors use it as an umbrella, and it causes the Sécurité Sociale [National Health Insurance] a tremendous cost, and maybe only one woman in 100,000 is helped." Doing lipid "profiles" on all candidates for the pill was probably the reason that, in a survey of French health, four times more persons said they had problems with lipid metabolism in 1980 than in 1970.

In the 1970s, at a time when the IUD was being freely prescribed to women in the United States whether or not they had had children, most French doctors were emphasizing that IUDs should not be used in women who had not had children (they usually specified at least two) because of the danger of pelvic inflammatory disease and, as a consequence, sterility. American gynecologists accepted this point of view much more slowly, requiring first a study that showed that IUDs increased the risk of pelvic inflammatory disease, then studies that showed it increased the risk of sterility—although most people knew that pelvic inflammatory disease increased the risk of sterility. By 1985, when a good number of U.S. gynecologists were ready to limit the use of IUDs to women with children, the issue was out of their hands—most IUDs were being taken off the market because so many women whose fertility had been damaged by them were suing.

French women don't make much use of the diaphragm, either. According to a 1977 study of married women of reproductive age using any form of contraception, only 2 percent used any female barrier method, including diaphragms, spermicides, and cervical caps, compared to 10 percent of American women. "French women always make a face when you mention a diaphragm," said Professor Netter. "They are very hostile to it, they don't like it, they find it inelegant." Some American women, however, who asked their French doctors for diaphragms, found it was the doctors who didn't like them. The diaphragm's failure to become a popular method of birth control in France may have to do with the fact that until recently, the diaphragm, like all forms of contraception, was illegal in France. By the time the ban was lifted, the pill was on the market; thus the diaphragm has no history in France.

One French answer to contraception is not what the woman does but what the man does: withdraw. According to the World Fertility Survey of the late 1970s, 29 percent of married French women of reproductive age used this method, almost as many as the 34 percent who used the pill. While withdrawal was not as common in France as it was in Bulgaria (79 percent), Czechoslovakia (31 percent), Italy (46 percent), Romania (44 percent), and Spain (44 percent), it was much more common in France than in Britain (6 percent) and the United States (3 percent). According to Sanche de Gramont, "The traditional advice of a mother to her daughter is: 'It is up to your husband to be careful.' As one French wife put it: 'It's like a meal where you've had plenty to eat and you're very pleased even though there is no dessert.' "

Another French practice shaped by concern over fertility is the reluctance of French doctors to perform hysterectomy in young women. Exact figures on the number of hysterectomies performed in France are impossible to obtain, but every indication shows the rate to be much lower than that in the United States, perhaps one-third. Dr. Thérèse Lecomte of the medical economy division of CREDOC, a social science research organization in Paris, found in one household survey that 2.4 percent of *all* French women reported having had a hysterectomy. This included women of all ages and would certainly be higher if only the older age groups were considered, but it is certainly lower than in the United States, where 1 percent of women ages 25 to 34, and 2 percent of women 35 to 44 have hysterectomies *each year.* Other comparisons have shown that the proportion of hysterectomized women in France is lower than that in England, and the English hysterectomy rate is not even one-half the U.S. rate.

While U.S. gynecologists give a wide range of reasons to perform hysterectomy, including sterilization and elimination of menstrual bleeding, most French gynecologists say there are only two indications in young women: cancer, and abnormal uterine bleeding that cannot be controlled in any other way. French medical texts suggest that myomectomy (removal of fibroid tumors with preservation of the uterus) is the treatment of choice for fibroids in women under forty, whereas only the most liberal texts in the United States suggest this for women *if* continued childbearing is desired. My own experience with fibroids in France was that hysterectomy was not even mentioned as an option for fibroid tumors. Since I was thirty-three, the doctor said, and I could still have children, I should have the myomectomy then to avoid a hysterectomy later.

Professor Netter, admitting that he was giving a very rough estimate, suggested that, at least in the university medical schools, approximately 70 percent of younger women with fibroids would have myomectomies and 30 percent hysterectomies. By contrast, myomectomies have been so rarely performed in the United States that many women have never heard of the operation: more myomectomies are being performed recently, however, based partly on the European experience and consumer demand.

Dr. Netter suggested that this greater tendency to conserve the uterus is due to two factors: the greater desire of French women to keep their uteruses and the separation of gynecologic surgery from obstetrics in France.

Until recently, he said, "obstetrics was always considered an inferior speciality," Dr. Netter said, noting that there was an old saying that if your son is clever, he should go into medicine; if good with his hands, into surgery; and if a little dull, into obstetrics. With a special corps of gynecologic surgeons who had the time (because they were not delivering babies) to develop finer skills, the myomectomy came into favor. "Gynecologic surgeons, to distinguish themselves from obstetricians, liked the operation of myomectomy because it was difficult and delicate—not everybody could do it."

He also suggested that the prevalence of hysterectomy in the United States was due to the all-or-nothing ideology there.

Traditionally, if French surgeons did perform a hysterectomy they did the "subtotal," that is, one that left in the uterine cervix. They cited the role of the cervix in maintaining the stability of the pelvic floor as well as sexual responsiveness.

Until very recently these reasons were pooh-poohed in England, West Germany, and the United States, partly because a New York surgeon in the 1940s had compared the two operations and found an equally high rate of loss of sexual responsiveness following both types. One German surgeon told me the subtotal would be considered malpractice in West Germany, and most medical insurers in the United States will not cover it.

British health consumer advocate Jean Robinson, after reading *La Nouvelle Presse Médicale*, asked her doctor: "What about a subtotal?" She was told, "I wouldn't be doing my best for you."

"He was astonished that anyone should question, and I was told that nobody does subtotals nowadays," said Mrs. Robinson, who nevertheless found an older gynecologist to perform her subtotal in the presence of medical students.

But very recently reports have begun to show that the French may have been right all along. A study in Finland demonstrated that the frequency of orgasms decreased significantly in women undergoing total hysterectomy, in contrast to the group who underwent subtotal hysterectomy, where the number of orgasms decreased, but not in statistically significant numbers.

Men, too, are likely to find that their sexual and reproductive organs are treated more gently in France than elsewhere. In the United States, for example, cancer of the prostate is often treated by prostatectomy and castration. In France, it is more likely to be treated by radiation therapy and low-dose estrogens or chemotherapy instead of castration. The radiation therapy has fewer complications than does the surgical treatment used in the United States, according to Dr. Jean-Pierre Armand, a cancer specialist at the Institut Gustave Roussy near Paris. Endocrinologist Dr. Philippe Bouchard added: "I think the fact that castration is performed less often in France may have something to do with the fact that it is a Catholic country."

Many cancers in France are treated with radiotherapy, perhaps because radiotherapists have traditionally enjoyed a very high prestige in France, the country where Marie and Pierre Curie did their work on radium. Cancer specialists in France have traditionally been radiotherapists, and not only prostate cancer but breast, skin, and uterine cancer are commonly treated by radiotherapy. But while tradition may be one reason for the widespread use of radiotherapy, this treatment often gives a better cosmetic result than surgery, and the French. in general, highly value good cosmetic results.

For it is not only in the treatment of breast cancer that sexuality, aesthetics, and psychology play a greater role in the way a French doctor weighs the risks and benefits of treatment than in the way his counterparts elsewhere do; such values are taken seriously in all aspects of medicine.

The importance of aesthetics can be seen in everything from how the French view artificial limbs to the way they ensure that women have at least ten free physical therapy sessions for getting into shape after giving birth. The French gave us the concept of *cellulite* (which has nothing to do with its dictionary definition of cellulitis but refers to that particularly female form of fat that deposits on the thighs and upper arms) and several ways to treat it. They also gave us the aesthetic surgeon Paul Tessier, whose total remodeling of the faces of severely deformed individuals revolutionized aesthetic surgery. Recently, French researchers reported a less radical technique for treating cancer of the penis that reconstructed the glans and allowed for a better aesthetic result.

The French focus on aesthetics seems to be shared with other Latin countries. Dr. Jean Pillet of Paris, discussing whether a patient missing a hand should be given a functional or a cosmetically good prosthesis, said that most of his patients who want a cosmetic device are from southern countries, with few from northern countries such as West Germany or England. "The Latin patients seem to feel they are not whole as a person after the amputation of a hand or a finger," he said. "It is important for them to have a complete body. But people from the northern countries don't have the same feelings. They are more interested in being functional than aesthetically pleasing." A contact-lens salesman interviewed in the mid-1970s said that the same was true for contact lenses, with Italy probably having the highest per capita use of contact lenses and England being a rather poor market. "In the United States," said Dr. Vladmir Mitz, a Parisian plastic surgeon, "people want plastic surgery [in order] to be rich. In France, they want it to be happy. In Sweden, you are supposed to be satisfied with your body as it is."

Whether the French undergo more cosmetic surgery than the Germans, English, and Americans cannot be known, since there are no French figures on such operations. But plastic surgeons familiar with France and America report a striking difference in the types of operations performed. Americans want their faces lifted while the French want the fat chiseled away from their abdomen, hips, and thighs in the procedure known as body sculpting. And while most Americans who undergo breast surgery want their breasts *enlarged*, French women, living in a country where the fashion industry has always been somewhat anti-bosom, want theirs *reduced*. In both countries these operations can sometimes be obtained for "medical" reasons.

The figures from the United States are clear, or nearly so. A survey of worldwide membership in the American Society of Plastic and Reconstructive Surgery (most of whose members are from the United States) showed that breast augmentations were performed twice as often as breast reductions. French surgeons interviewed, on the other hand, indicate that breast reduction is at least three to four times more common than breast augmentation. Dr. Mitz estimated that in France surgeons do roughly eight reductions for every two augmentations. Similar figures were given by Dr. Denys Montandon of Geneva, in the French-speaking part of Switzerland.

This has nothing to do with French women being larger and needing more reduction, a fact that can be verified by checking out bra sizes in the department stores: The large sizes common in U.S. stores are practically unknown in France. Rather, it has to do with what constitutes an ideal body size.

"An American woman must have large breasts," said Dr. Mitz. "If we're talking in terms of meat, the ideal breast in France would weigh 250 grams [8.8 ounces], in the United States 400 grams [14 ounces]. The ideal bust measurement in France would be 85 centimeters [33 inches] and that in America 100 centimeters [39 inches]." To achieve this ideal, he said, American plastic surgeons usually use a prosthesis about one and one half times the size of that used in France in the rare case when augmentation is even considered. "Many breasts reduced in France would be considered very beautiful in America," he said.

Another striking difference is the prevalence of face-lifts, the sixth most common cosmetic procedure in the United States. "When I worked in the United States," Dr. Mitz said, "we did about one 'lifting' a day. Here, we do one 'lifting' every two weeks." In France, he explained, "to age is to enter into a social category that has its place. When people do get face-lifts, they usually do so either to continue to work, or because their children tell them to."

The French concern with thinness may seem paradoxical in light of the French preoccupation with food. But it's not the quantity of food eaten that distinguishes France from the rest of the world: it's the care taken with the quality and character of what's eaten.

Medically, this has several consequences. One seems to be that lack of appetite is a more serious symptom for a Frenchman than it would be, say, for an Englishman. Indeed, one young French doctor recalls being taught in medical school that it was a sign of cancer. Lack of appetite is less important for a Swede or an Englishman, said Dr. Göran Kielberg of the Department of Social Medicine at the University Hospital of Uppsala. "If you told an English doctor that you'd lost your appetite, he'd say, 'So what?' "

French eating and drinking habits, in fact, may explain why the French have the longest life spans of the four countries under study. While they do have the highest rates of cirrhosis in the world, they also have (if statistics can be believed) a much lower incidence of heart attack, 100 per 100,000 population, compared to 240 in West Germany, 300 in the United States, and 350 in the United Kingdom. Even when French men were matched for the risk factors of hypertension, diabetes, high cholesterol, and smoking with men from Framingham, Massachusetts, the French were less likely than the Framingham men to have heart attacks: A Frenchman's risk at fifty corresponds to that of an American male at forty, Dr. Jacques-Lucien Richard reported at a press conference held by the Institut National de la Santé et de la Recherche Médicale. Since moderate drinking has been found to correlate with a lesser risk of heart attack, some doctors speculate that French drinking habits may at least partially protect them from the high rates of heart attacks found elsewhere.

But eating well, many French people believe, is responsible for what for many years was the national pathology, the liver crisis, or *crise de foie*.

While Americans acknowledge their livers only when they have hepatitis or a full-fledged cirrhosis, the French are acutely aware of theirs every time they eat. One well-known French advertisement for mineral water asks a gourmand about to de-

vour huge quantities of rich food: "And your liver?" The gourmand replies: "My liver doesn't know," implying that the mineral
water being advertised so protects the liver that the food will
have no ill effects.

French doctors examine the liver more often than do British
doctors, and the French firmly believe that eating rich food
causes liver problems. One British GP who spent a week ob-
serving a French country doctor tells of a farmer's son, age ten,
with an enlarged liver that the doctor attributed to overeating,
presumably in the same way that geese in a farmyard produce
foie gras.

French patients and their doctors attribute an extremely wide
variety of complaints in other parts of their bodies to their livers,
according to Dr. Claude Béraud, a professor of hepatology and
gastroenterology at the University of Bordeaux in his 1983 book,
Le Foie des Français. The diagnosis of *crise de foie* is usually given
to what in reality is a migraine headache: Dr. Béraud says that
migraines account for 80 percent of French liver crises.

"Nine of ten French patients believe that their headaches are
due to the liver," agreed another liver specialist, Dr. Jean-Pierre
Benhamou, a professor of gastroenterology at Hôpital Beaujon
in the Parisian suburbs. "The French patient says he has *mal
aux reins* (pain in the kidneys) when he really has backache;
he says he has *mal au coeur* (pain in the heart) when he wants
to vomit. He doesn't believe that either the kidneys or the heart
are to blame. When, however, he talks of the *crise de foie,* he
really does believe it's the liver."

Most of the *crises de foie* that aren't migraines, according to
Dr. Béraud, are gastrointestinal upsets of one kind or another.

But the liver is held responsible for complaints more subtle
than the acute *crise.* According to Dr. Béraud, French people
and their doctors attribute an extremely wide range of complaints to the liver, including painful menstruation, paleness,
yellowness, and general fatigue. Both patients and dermatologists sometimes accuse the liver of causing acne or rash, dan-
druff, herpes, and other skin complaints.

"For ear-nose-and-throat specialists, the liver causes rhinitis and tonsillitis and pharyngitis," Dr. Béraud wrote. "Chest specialists and allergists sometimes say the liver is responsible for allergic reactions such as asthma or hay fever." Dr. Béraud claims he found a description of "hereditary hepatism," and tonsillitis and sore throats of "hepatic origin" on mimeographed sheets going to medical students in 1969.

But that isn't all, writes Dr. Béraud. Mothers explain the laziness of their children by a "hepatic" temperament, and motion sickness is thought by some to be due to the liver. The organ is also held responsible for some nervous depressions, palpitations, low blood pressure, insomnia, and faints. Dr. Béraud even cited the thirty-seven-year-old executive patient who thought his impotence must be due to the liver, and the highly educated young woman who felt her persistent cough was due to an enlarged liver that inhibited her breathing.

The origins of the French concern about the liver are unknown: Dr. Henri Pequignot suggested that it dates back at least to medieval times. Dr. Béraud says that the diagnosis of "minor hepatic insufficiency"—supposedly the failure of the liver to produce adequate bile—originated around 1880 and became popular in the first half of the twentieth century, encouraged by both the spa towns and the newly developing pharmaceutical industry. Between 1920 and 1950, he said, French radiologists and gastroenterologists invented "a great quantity of details and of falsely scientific explanation to respond to the demand of patients and general practitioners, a little like a cookie maker diversifying his product in response to demand created by a well-carried-out advertising campaign."

"The *crise de foie* reinforces the social significance of the act of eating and drinking in France," wrote a Princeton University student who studied the *crise de foie* for her thesis. "It signifies the superior quality of the French meal, and the pride the French feel in that high quality."

One of the explanations advanced for patients' symptoms was biliary dyskinesia, or abnormal motion of the bile duct.

There are many types of such dyskinesias, according to the "Godeau," the basic French textbook of internal medicine. A bile duct may have normal tone (*normotonique*) but too much movement (*hypercinétique*), with a normal volume at fasting but a too rapid evacuation. According to the "Godeau," a bile duct may be both *hypertonique* and *hypercinétique*, or *normotonique* but *hypocinétique*, or *hypotonique* and *hypocinétique*. According to Dr. Béraud, these diagnoses resulted when a patient complaining of a liver crisis was sent for an X ray of his bile duct and no stones were found: rather than tell a patient there was nothing wrong, he would be told either that the bile duct emptied too quickly or that it didn't empty quickly enough. The pharmaceutical industry then started making drugs to fit the diagnoses: *cholérétiques*, to increase bile secretion; *cholécysto-kinétiques*, supposed to contract the bile duct, and *antispasmo-diques*, to reduce bile secretion.

In 1970, there were three hundred different drugs for the liver in France, accounting for nearly 5 percent of French drug consumption. A comparison between French and American drug consumption in 1976 showed that 12 percent of French drugs, compared to 5 percent of U.S. drugs, were for the digestive system. The difference is even more striking when one realizes that French per-capita drug consumption is greater overall than that in the United States.

In 1976, French hepatologists held a press conference absolving the liver of its responsibility for most diseases (except, of course, cirrhosis and hepatitis), and since then it has been unfashionable to talk about the *crise de foie*, although one still hears about bile ducts. The medical economy division of the Centre de Recherches et de Documentation sur la Consommation (CREDOC) found that between 1970 and 1980 the number of persons saying that they suffered from liver disease declined by a factor of four. The sale of drugs for the liver also seems to have dropped dramatically: the 1982 study of prescriptions for the Office of Health Economics in London found a relative excess of gastrointestinal drugs for Italy but not for France.

But echoes of the French concern about the liver can still be heard in France and perhaps even the world:

- Nearly 7.5 percent of French drugs, everything from aspirin to antibiotics, comes as suppositories, compared to about 1 percent in the United States. While this may be related to the French predilection for taking temperatures rectally, one visiting English doctor was told that the reason for so many suppositories was that drugs absorbed through the rectum do not pass through the liver.
- While a common anemia in England or America would probably be treated by iron, in France the patient is as likely to receive either a prescription for vitamin B_{12}, a vitamin originally isolated from liver extracts, or a prescription for liver extracts themselves. While vitamin B_{12} is the proper treatment for pernicious anemia, a rare disease, in France B_{12} is widely used for practically any anemia. According to Dr. Jacques Messerschmitt in his book *La Médecine contre la santé*, the extremely important role of the liver in French medical culture undoubtedly set the stage for the extremely loose indications for the liver vitamin, which the pharmaceutical industry in France used to its advantage.
- In 1980, a French drug, Selacryn, which had been recently approved for the treatment of hypertension in the United States after several years of use in France, was withdrawn from the U.S. market after twenty-four deaths and 363 cases of liver damage were ascribed to it. The French knew that the drug had side effects, although they didn't regard them as serious. However, the French system for identifying side effects of drugs, which is acknowledged to be a good system, was handicapped in this case because such a system "demands an acute awareness of drugs as a possible cause of certain conditions when they first present." While an American patient and doctor would immediately suspect a drug if liver complications developed, French patients, many of whom have

been told all their lives that they have "fragile livers," probably would not.

The concept that some people have a "fragile liver" or "fragile bile duct," as opposed to one simply overwhelmed by excess food and drink, illustrates another major characteristic of French medicine: the importance of the *terrain*. There is no really good translation for *terrain* in English. The old-fashioned word "constitution," which has largely gone out of favor in America, probably translates it best. "Risk factors" can describe aspects of the *terrain* but connotes particular aspects, whereas *terrain* is a more all-encompassing concept. "Resistance" used in a general sense is also close to the meaning, but "resistance" is usually used in the specific sense of resistance to a specific disease, and that is not at all what *terrain* means. Many diseases result from a combination of some type of outside insult and the body's reaction to that insult. While English and American doctors tend to focus on the insult, the French and Germans focus on the reaction and are more likely to try to find ways to modify the reaction as well as fight off the insult.

One American medical historian recounted what happened when he saw a French doctor after a couple of his toenails fell off. While the medical historian (and the Australian doctor he eventually saw) felt the problem had arisen because his sneakers were too tight, the French doctor discounted the role of the environment, in this case sneakers. Instead, he claimed something was out of balance in the historian's body and prescribed months of calcium and magnesium therapy.

Even Louis Pasteur, who is regarded as the father of modern microbiology, accorded an importance to the *terrain* at least equal to the specific microbe. The late Dr. René Dubos, himself a proselytizer for the importance of *terrain*, spoke of Pasteur's views during a colloquium commemorating the one hundred fiftieth anniversary of the birth of Pasteur. "He even went as far as to suggest that the psychologic state could influence resistance to microbes," Dr. Dubos said, quoting from Pasteur: " 'How many times does the constitution of the injured, his weakening, his morale . . . set up a barrier to the invasion of the infinitely tiny organisms that is insufficient.' "

Focus on the *terrain* shapes French medicine in a number of ways. It skews drug consumption away from antibiotics, which fit the English and American concept of disease as invader, toward tonics, vitamins, and "modifiers of the *terrain*" and more recently, toward ways to stimulate the immune system. It favors treatments such as rest and stays at France's spas as ways to build up the *terrain*. It favors fringe medicines such as home-opathy and aromatherapy. It makes the French leaders in fields that concentrate on shoring up the *terrain*, such as immuno-therapy for cancer. And it results in a decidedly more casual attitude toward the elimination of dirt and germs than that seen in many other countries.

Spasmophilia, a uniquely French diagnosis that increased sevenfold between 1970 and 1980, is an interesting case history of how French medicine views *terrain*. "I've seen thousands of cases here," said Dr. Jean Durlach of France about spasmophilia, "and I think about six cases have been reported in the American medical literature."

Both Dr. Durlach, and the late Dr. Henri-Pierre Klotz, the Parisian professor who first defined "adult spasmophilia" in 1948, admitted that the French do not differ in any way phys-iologically from the Americans and English. "It's cultural," said Dr. Durlach, who explained that the two tests crucial to a di-agnosis of spasmophilia, Chvostek's sign and electromyography, are simply not done in North America, at least not in the normal medical consultation. Chvostek's sign is a reflex provoked by tapping the face on a line going from the outer lip to the ear: if the lips puff out, which occurs in about 14 percent of patients, the sign is considered positive, according to Dr. Klotz. If the sign is positive, the patient may be referred for an electromyographic examination. If a repetitive pattern is found, the patient is di-agnosed a *spasmophile*. According to the last published *Journée*

du K, electromyography, in search of either normality or spasmophilia, was the twenty-ninth most commonly performed procedure in France: on November 30, 1982, taken to be a typical
day of medical practice, the diagnosis of spasmophilia was as
frequent as that of hearing problems.

But what is spasmophilia? The technical term is that it is
latent, normocalcemic tetany (tetany is a state of muscular spasms
seen, for example, in hyperventilation syndrome), and Dr. Durlach adds the qualifications constitutional and idiopathic (of
unknown cause). A clearer definition would be a *tendency* to
hyperventilation syndrome, even though you can be a spasmophile without actually having hyperventilated. Dr. Klotz noted
that anyone can become tetanic after hyperventilating for a long
enough time, while spasmophiles generally become tetanic after
just a few minutes of hyperventilation. In other words, it's the
terrain that predisposes to hyperventilation.

Spasmophilia probably corresponds most closely to chronic
hyperventilation syndrome, a syndrome described in the English-language literature but not commonly diagnosed. The various symptoms—anxiety, fatigue, headache, dizziness, cramps,
cardiac palpitations, extrasystole, mitral valve prolapse—are
common to both the diseases, as is the tendency to hyperven-
tilate. But the conditions are diagnosed and treated in entirely
different ways. While in England one would at least need symptoms, including probably at least one instance of hyperventilation, to receive a diagnosis of chronic hyperventilation syndrome,
in France merely meeting the criteria of the positive Chvostek's
sign and abnormal electromyography would be enough to be
labeled a spasmophile for life.

Chronic hyperventilation syndrome in England is treated by
teaching the patient how to slow down his breathing, and acute
hyperventilation syndrome is treated by having him breathe into
a paper bag (to increase the amount of carbon dioxide in the
blood). In France, spasmophilia is treated by either vitamin D
or magnesium, and hyperventilation is treated by an intravenous injection of calcium, which causes an immediate sense of

well-being. "A British doctor would be very skeptical about giving an injection to treat this condition," said Dr. Mark Ball, a British psychiatrist practicing in Hannover, West Germany, when told about French spasmophilia. "It creates dependence on a medical person to give the injection. The British doctor, who is not paid on a fee-for-service basis, has a vested interest in keeping the patient as independent as possible."

Dr. Durlach strongly believes spasmophilia is caused by magnesium deficiency. In any case, he says, the magnesium cannot hurt anyone, since most people's magnesium intake is marginal and any excess is eliminated in the urine. Dr. F. M. Hull, an English GP who noted the large number of prescriptions for magnesium in a day spent with a French doctor, suggested that the magnesium is probably acting like milk of magnesia—as a laxative.

"They used to call Frenchmen frog-eaters—now they call us magnesium eaters," said Dr. Klotz, who believed the condition is due to an abnormality of calcium metabolism that should be treated with vitamin D, if at all. Dr. Klotz, shortly before his death in 1984, was somewhat aghast at the use being made of his diagnosis. Some French doctors, for example, have written books promoting spasmophilia as a lifelong illness nothing short of catastrophic; and the diagnosis is often made casually, raising the number of spasmophiles way above its already high 14 percent of the population. While Dr. Klotz did believe spasmophiles might need special treatment during pregnancy and following psychological or physiological shock, he admitted that most spasmophiles might be better off living in England, where the condition is not recognized.

But perhaps not in America. A French translator working in Washington suffered fainting spells, for which she was hospitalized and given multiple uncomfortable tests that ultimately found nothing. She returned to France, was immediately labeled a spasmophile, started taking magnesium, and has felt fine ever since.

The belief in the importance of the *terrain* strongly influences not only diagnosis but also French drug use. If the *terrain* is more important than the disease, it becomes less important to fight the disease "aggressively" and more important to shore up the *terrain*. While American doctors love to use the word "aggressive," the French much prefer *les médecines douces*, or "gentle therapies."

In the United States, it is rare for an M.D. to use "fringe medicine." In France it is not. Take for example homeopathy, a system based on the fact that people have different *terrains* and that smaller doses are more powerful than larger ones. According to a survey done in 1978, six thousand French doctors prescribed homeopathic treatments, with about half of these using homeopathy exclusively. Of the pharmacists sampled, 55 percent recommended homeopathic treatments occasionally and the vast majority thought that homeopathic treatments would increase in the future. When François Mitterrand was elected president of France, he decreed that such therapies were worthy of further study, and in recent years the popularity of homeopathy has mushroomed.

A 1984 *Guide pratique des médecines douces* listed twenty-eight different types of gentle medicines, not counting *cellulothérapie, gemmothérapie, isothérapie* (using remedies made from the patient's own secretions in homeopathic dilutions), *lithothérapie, micro-minéralothérapie, mycothérapie, opothérapie,* and *organothérapie,* which were grouped together under the heading of biotherapies. The French even developed a practice appropriate to a country known for its perfume industry—a practice called aromatherapy, where the inhalation of various scents is said to have a healing effect. While mainstream doctors sometimes use an antibiogram in order to determine the sensitivity of a germ to various antibiotics, doctors practicing aromatherapy use aromatograms to determine the antibiotic action of several plants in relation to the *terrain* of the patient. As for drugs and therapies of mainstream medicine in France, those meant to fight germs play a lesser role, and those aimed at modifying the *terrain* play a greater role, than they would in England or America. By the same token, antibiotics occupy a less important role in total drug use in France.

In a 1976 CREDOC comparison of French and American drug use, such tonics and "modifiers of the *terrain*" accounted for 10.1 percent of drugs prescribed in France, compared to 3.7 percent in the United States. In the 1982 data provided by the British Office of Health Economics study, there were as many prescriptions for tonics in France as there were for broad-spectrum penicillins—and no other classes of antibiotics even made the list of the twenty most commonly prescribed classes of drugs. By contrast, in the United Kingdom, no tonics made the top twenty, but broad-spectrum penicillins ranked seventh in frequency, tetracyclines ranked twelfth, and medium- and narrow-spectrum penicillins ranked sixteenth.

The French preference for gentle therapies also affects the dosage prescribed of mainstream drugs; generally it is smaller and treatments are less aggressive than in the United States. This applies to drugs of proven efficacy: researchers on the blood thinner urokinase, for example, speak of the "French dose," which is half the "American dose," and recommended doses of the pain-killer paracetamol are less than half those in the United States and Britain. Even the strongest types of drugs may be weaker in France. The shah of Iran was prescribed chlorambucil for his cancer by his French doctors, and American doctors were surprised that he had not been given a stronger drug.

A belief in the *terrain* also undoubtedly plays a role in the fact that fewer invasive procedures are used in intensive care units in France than in the United States—with patients doing equally well in both countries.

Another consequence is more limited operations. The propensity for myomectomy, subtotal hysterectomy, and lesser operations for prostate cancer has already been mentioned, but other procedures are also affected. French doctors do not believe in routine circumcision of newborn males, for example, but occasionally they perform the procedure for religious reasons, or, for Americans, for "hygienic" ones. But "French" circumcision is not identical to American circumcision, as more of the prepuce is left intact.

The belief in the importance of the *terrain* explains at least in part French attitudes to dirt and to germs in general. The French see a little bit of dirt not as the enemy, but as being good for the *terrain* and worth cultivating.

The English and Americans have a saying, "Cleanliness is next to godliness." The French don't. While Americans assume that if it's clean it must be healthy, the French are quick to point out the health advantages of dirt, or at least the health advantages of tolerating dirt.

One famous French surgeon of earlier decades reportedly said that in French hospital practice clean knees are an index of moral frailty (whether he meant the patient's or the staff's knees is unclear). A 1976 article in *Le Monde* about French legal rights pointed out that while the French hospital patient has the right to keep his clothes, refuse operation, and have his family doctor come, he doesn't have the right to a bath once a week. "The rules specify only a monthly bath. Only feet washing is weekly." While American deodorant advertisements emphasize how dry their product makes you, French deodorants advertise, "You have the right to perspire" (antiperspirants in France don't "stop" perspiration, they "regulate" it). When feminine deodorants came out, French consumer groups not only repeated the American argument that they could be dangerous to one's health but added that the deodorants eliminated smells necessary for sexual attraction. Napoleon reportedly wrote his wife Josephine, "Don't bathe, I'm coming home." The French use an average of 4.2 bars of soap per person per year, compared to 8.3 in England.

"The French don't believe in soap and water," said Dr. R. S. Inch, an English doctor working for a pharmaceutical firm in France. "For some things they're quite right. Americans, by showering and washing, remove essential oils, which does cause aging."

For many years French dermatologists have advised people

not to wash their hair and skin too much. This is not surprising for persons with dry hair and skin, and American dermatologists would probably advise the same. What makes the French advice different is that people with oily hair are also told not to wash it more than once a week, if possible.

Many French doctors believe that washing oily hair simply causes greater amounts of oil to be secreted. This doctrine is known as reactive seborrhea, and has been popularized by Dr. R. Aron-Brunetière in his book, *La Beauté et la médecine*. Dr. Aron-Brunetière also counsels people with oily skin to avoid washing it at all with soap and water, while such washing has been the mainstay of the American dermatologists' advice. According to the *AMA Book of Skin and Hair Care*, "Most physicians recommend that their acne patients wash several times a day."

Dry hair, oily hair, and acne are not the only problems that lie in wait for those too eager to cleanse themselves, in the French opinion. In 1977, a study in *Le Concours médical* concluded that frequent shampooing with detergent shampoos was responsible for hair loss in women.

The French also warn about too much cleanliness in restaurants, food places, water supplies, and toilet seats. Some foods that meet French standards of sterilization, certain *foie gras*, for example, cannot necessarily be sold in the United States.

"There is no fight against germs here," said Professor Jacques Acar of Hôpital Saint-Jacques in Paris. "There's a tolerance for them." According to Dr. Acar, "If someone gets sick after a banquet, they know it's the food, but there's a tolerance for the germ, especially if the disease is not serious. Even serious infections are not taken that seriously."

The late Cornelius Kruse, Ph.D., a sanitary engineer, of the Johns Hopkins School of Public Health, said that during World War II he had been in charge of securing clean water supplies for Allied troups in Europe. When he wanted to chlorinate the supply of a small French town, the mayor objected, saying, "But that would be like putting a brassiere on the Vénus de Milo." Dr. Kruse added, "I get the idea that every country that was under the French colonial system is chaotic where it concerns public health. There is always a relaxed attitude. In the ex-British colonies, there was always a public water supply that worked halfway well, with sanitarians and health inspectors."

"The human organism is made to defend itself," said Dr. Gilbert Martin-Bouyer, chief of the Transmissible Disease Section of the Institut National de la Santé et de la Recherche Médicale, who became practically livid when I brought up the question of restaurant inspections, particularly whether dirty toilets weren't a public health concern. "Name me one disease transmitted by toilet seats," he challenged. A French doctor friend agreed, promising he would take me to dinner if I could come up with the answer.

Besides feeling that excessive worry about dirt diverts energies that could be more productively used elsewhere, many French doctors cite a number of diseases, such as *turista* and allergies and serious consequences of hepatitis A and toxoplasmosis, they believe they are avoiding by their greater exposure to dirt. Dr. Georges Halpern, an allergist living in Paris, believes the French may have fewer allergies because of "our dirty way of life here," noting that he fed his infant children exactly the same food he and his wife ate. The French also don't get *turista* when they travel, according to one French doctor, because they've acquired the immunity at home.

A dirty life-style can also allow exposure to certain germs, a form of natural vaccination that the French tend to favor over man's vaccinations. Exposure to certain germs earlier in life can lead to less severe results. Hepatitis A, for example, is a fairly mild disease when it occurs in childhood, but a more serious disease in adults. Eighty to 90 percent of persons forty years of age and older in France have antibody to hepatitis A, meaning that they have had the disease whether they knew it or not. The comparable figure in Sweden is 50 percent, with 50 percent of the population still at risk, meaning that Swedes on the average get hepatitis at an older age and are probably more severely affected.

Still another disease that is less harmful the sooner it's contracted is toxoplasmosis. Toxoplasmosis, like rubella, is dangerous only when acquired during pregnancy, when it can cause
birth defects in the fetus. French women have usually acquired
the disease before they reach childbearing age due to the French
habit of eating undercooked meat. Women who do have problems with toxoplasmosis in France are usually immigrants who
took up French habits at about the same time they became
pregnant.

Still another aspect of *terrain* is the French emphasis on rest,
sick leaves, and spas. The French have the legal right to five
weeks of vacation a year and no French man or woman would
dream of not taking it. Frenchmen have been known to refuse
high government appointments because it interfered with their
vacations. If five weeks is considered necessary for a healthy
person to recuperate from a year's work, it should not be surprising that French hospital stays have typically been about
twice those in the United States for the same procedures. While
hospital stays have been falling in all countries in recent years,
there is resistance from the French people to short stays. In
1981, the average length of stay in obstetric and gynecology
services of French public hospitals was 6.7 days, in maternity
hospitals with operating rooms 8 days, and in maternity hospitals without operating rooms 10.6 days. When French women
were asked if they would like to leave the hospital twenty-four
hours after giving birth if everything went well and if house
calls and household help were provided, 61 percent of pregnant
women and 72 percent of those who had recently given birth
were opposed. The majority of pregnant women wanted to stay
in the hospital a week or more, and those who had recently
given birth thought five to six days was ideal.

French sick leaves are so long and are taken so often that
they often become a joke among foreigners in France. Dr. Jacques
Messerschmitt recounts the case of a woman who had been on
sick leave for six and a half years for a "gynecologic anemia"
that had never been very severe.

The belief in rest was defended by one French tuberculosis expert at a meeting where it had been pointed out that English, Dutch, and American studies had shown that rest did absolutely nothing for TB. "If we ask our body to defend itself against an infection such as tuberculosis, it will be better able to do it if we give it rest and sufficient nutrition instead of continuing to submit it to important efforts such as work. And especially if this active life takes place in the more and more polluted atmosphere of our large cities."

While long hospital stays, sick leaves, and "sleep cures" for psychiatric illness are favored in France, it is considered even better if you can get out of the city to take the *cure* at one of France's ninety-six approved spas.

The idea that city life is unhealthy was promulgated by the philosophers Jean-Jacques Rousseau, Sébastien Mercier, and Restif de la Bretonne, among others, said Claudine Herzlich, a medical sociologist at the Ecoles Pratiques des Hautes Etudes in Paris. "The idea of the unhealthy character of the city spread," she said, "and continues in France." Sherry Turkle suggests in *Psychoanalytic Politics* that French nostalgia for a simpler way of life affected the development of French psychiatry. "Even as the stability of French rural society was in the process of crumbling, French psychiatry continued to express its nostalgia for a simpler, more rooted life in the provinces," Turkle writes. "French psychiatric studies spoke of the pathology inherent in urban life and warned that leaving 'organic and alive' rural settings for 'artificial' urban ones would have only the most deleterious effects on mental health . . . by taking [this position] and expressing it in what was often a passionate rhetoric, French psychiatry served to bolster a social ideology that glorified rural life and traditional values."

One in every two hundred medical visits in France results in a prescription for the *cure*. After World War II the Sécurité Sociale decided to reimburse the costs of spa treatment in France, which caused the number of French people taking the *cure* to rise dramatically: in 1984, over half a million persons took the *cure*, with 95 percent of spa visits paid for at least in part by the health insurance. The French pride themselves in their "specialized" spas: persons suffering from rheumatic complaints may be sent to Aix-les-Bains; those suffering from liver complaints to Vichy, and those suffering from allergies may be sent to Le Mont-Doré. Ailments particularly amenable to spa treatment, according to a recent report to the French government, are arthritis, nose and throat problems, and bronchitis; some of the spas specializing in other ailments would like to change their specialization to these three categories. At the spa, where *curistes* must stay the full three weeks in order to be reimbursed, their spa doctor will write prescriptions for various treatments using the mineral waters and gases, prescribing the temperature and duration of treatment as well as what is to be done. The treatments are mostly either physical therapy carried out in thermal waters or washings of the various body orifices (enemas, douches, etc.). They often have elaborate names: At Aix-les-Bains, for example, one may be prescribed the Aix-Douche (a shower massage) or the Berthollet, in which warm air mixed with thermal vapor is applied to the affected joint or the whole body.

Spas, of course, are poohed-poohed in the United States and England and their effect is considered mostly psychosomatic. French spa doctors don't discount the fact that some of the good effects of spa treatment are psychosomatic, although they don't know what is so wrong with this. They do believe, however, that the good effects of spa treatments are more than psychosomatic, and indeed many treatments developed first in spas are also used outside the spas. Dr. François Besançon, a professor of spa medicine at the University of Paris, pointed out that Americans now heat the swimming pools in which they give physical therapy, which is just a step away from their use of naturally occurring hot springs.

One strong advocate of spas was the late Dr. Jacques Forestier, who received international fame for having been the first to use gold in rheumatoid arthritis and who introduced corticosteroid treatment to France. Dr. Forestier was a trim and lively eighty-two when I interviewed him in the mid-seventies and he told me, "You ought to try the *cure*—it's really something."

Dr. Forestier, who lived in Aix-les-Bains, said that he visited a particular spa each year as a patient, where he received treatment for a respiratory condition. Spas don't really cure you, he said, but they do produce a remission that lasts for eight to ten months—just in time to start getting ready for the next *cure*.

Commenting reflectively on the Anglo-Saxon disbelief in spas, he said: "It certainly shouldn't be said that they are behind us, it's simply a position they have taken. Medicine is not yet a very exact science, and there should still be room for many different points of view."

When I first went to France, I found many of these ideas backward; now, I find they make a good deal of sense. I have fiercely guarded my uterus in the face of U.S. medicine's belief that it should be removed; I have begun to attribute some of my headaches to my liver's inability to metabolize the amount of wine I am consuming; and I give more weight than I once did to aesthetic and pleasurable values when weighing the risks and benefits of medical treatment. I wash my face less often and find, in fact, my complexion has improved.

Perhaps most important, however, I have come to recognize the importance of the *terrain*. While I have not yet become an advocate of homeopathy, I believe in smaller doses unless a bigger dose has been proven better, and in refusing antibiotics unless they're *really* necessary. I no longer believe that an aggressive approach to disease is necessarily any better than a gentle one, and I no longer accept the statement that an aggressive disease takes an aggressive therapy: I want to know if the patient is actually better off with an aggressive therapy or a less aggressive one. For most of us, the *terrain* does work pretty well on its own, and a greater recognition of this in America would probably not hurt, and might even help, our medicine.

West Germany:
The Lingering Influences of Romanticism

He seems to value my mind and my various talents more than this heart of mine, of which I am so proud, for it is the source of all things—all strength, all bliss, all misery. The things I know, every man can know, but, oh, my heart is mine alone!
> —Johann Wolfgang von Goethe,
> *The Sorrows of Young Werther*

The heart is the key to the world.
> —Novalis

Even the most casual look at the current statistics on German drug use can be startling: West Germans use about six times the amount of heart drugs, per capita, as do the French and English.

It's not because there's more heart disease in West Germany. The French do have a lower rate of heart attacks, but the English do not. The death rate attributed to coronary artery disease in West Germany is actually lower than it is in England and the United States, and the death rate attributed to all types of heart disease is about the same in all three countries.

Why, then, such a huge consumption of heart drugs? Further probing offers two explanations. The seemingly excessive use of medication for the heart may be due, at least partly, to the widespread use of a diagnosis, *Herzinsuffizienz*, that is quite liberally applied without any corroborating evidence. In addition,

74

because Germans take a less mechanical view of the heart, people who would be treated by coronary artery bypass in the United States are treated by drugs in Germany.

When questioned as to why these and other medical traditions (such as a preoccupation with the circulation) flourished in West Germany and not elsewhere, several of my sources suggested that German romanticism had had something to do with it.

The literary, philosophical, and musical movement known as romanticism touched all of Europe to some extent in the nineteenth century, but the movement is most strongly associated with Germany. Romanticism is impossible to define precisely, but in many ways can be seen as the opposite of Cartesianism. Instead of valuing thought, romanticism values feeling, with unbounded faith in the life of the heart and the soul. Instead of viewing the world as a machine, as did the Cartesians, romantics viewed it as an organism. Romantic concepts of growth and development caused German scientists to take the lead in embryology: "The romantic anatomists and physiologists, being so greatly interested in embryology, were wont to use the microscope and to inquire into the genesis of tissues as well as of organic form," wrote medical historian Owsei Temkin.

Still another hallmark of romanticism was the notion of the synthesis or interplay of opposing forces. German philosophers such as Hegel and Marx developed explanations of the world based on thesis, antithesis, and synthesis; and German scientists developed explanations based on the interplay between positive and negative, attractive and repulsive, centripetal and centrifugal, expansile and contractile, oxidative and reductive, inner and outer, and male and female.

The basic concepts of this philosophy suffused the literature in nineteenth-century Germany, as well as in France, England, and America. "But upon English, French and American medicine their influence was nil," wrote the medical historian F. H.

Garrison. "Not so with the medicine of Southwestern Germany during 1800–1830"—where a movement known as romantic medicine flourished.

Germans no longer speak about romantic medicine. But much of their thinking about medicine seems to be determined by a romantic thought process that stems from their character and culture.

If you ask a non-German about the German character, you are apt to get a reply about someone who gives and follows orders. Dr. Mark Ball, a British psychiatrist practicing near Hannover, can see how an authoritarian attitude arises in West Germany. "Germans are very subservient to authority," he said. "The whole business of the civil service is extraordinary. It's a military system with ranks. The schools, universities, police force, and the administration are all governed this way. It's very difficult to complain. If you do, you must go through the various channels. The whole idea of *Berufsverboten*—that people with various beliefs could not serve in the civil service—was a way of showing that if you make a wrong step, there will be retribution."

Physicians in all countries tend to be authoritarian, but they may in fact be even more so in West Germany. When I asked German doctors what German patients usually think is wrong with them when they visit the doctor, they replied that German patients don't think anything because they have been taught it's not up to them to make the diagnosis.

But while outsiders focus on the authoritarian aspects of the German character, Germans themselves tend to see their chief characteristic as emotionalism. "Englishmen are not so emotional," said Professor Hans Schadewaldt of the Institute of the History of Medicine in Düsseldorf. "Italians are emotional and they show it; Germans are very emotional but they don't show it. Germans are more emotional than the French."

"Germans are terribly romantic, terribly abstract," said Felix Moos, Ph.D., a professor of anthropology at the University of Kansas in Lawrence, who grew up on the Swiss-German border.

Dr. Moos contrasted this with the American character, which he termed specific and particular. Germans, he said, are more holistic, tending to look at wholes rather than parts, and there is really no translation into English of their word *Gestalt*.

There is also no word that can adequately translate the German concept of *Geist*, or spirituality. While Americans often do things simply because they are practical, Dr. Moos said, "in Germany nothing is done without *Geist*. No German leader would ever allow the populace to believe he lacked *Geist*, and would tend to broadcast the fact that he listens to music and poetry." Medically this means, he said, that while Americans see the body as mechanical, Germans see health and the body as going hand in hand with *Geist* and nature. Part of the focus on balance that can be seen in German society, he believes, comes from the constant effort Germans have to make to balance that side of them that is efficient with their romantic side.

Germans also have the reputation for being pessimistic. While English fairy tales end "and they lived happily ever after," and the French add "and had lots of children," German fairy tales end, "and if they have not yet died they are still living." There is no word for "happy end" in German: in the rare case when Germans feel the concept is needed they borrow the English term and speak of *das Happy End*.

The West German health care system accommodates both the efficient and the romantic aspects of the German character by including both high-tech medicine, such as electrocardiograms and CAT scanners, and "soft" medicine based on the healing powers of nature, such as homeopathy and spas. The West German health care system, in fact, accommodates practically everything.

Doctors are reimbursed for what they do, whether they perform CAT scans or prescribe mud baths, and there is essentially little control on that as even the patients they do it to are not allowed to see the slips the German doctors send to the multiple health insurances detailing the procedures they have performed.

While German drug laws have tightened up somewhat since the thalidomide tragedies, only safety, not effectiveness, is required, and "everything is available here," said Dr. Karl Kimball, who is with a German doctors' drug group. There are 120,000 different drugs on the market in Germany, Dr. M. N. G. Dukes, then of the Dutch drug regulatory agency, informed me when I interviewed him, as compared to 1,180 in Iceland. He pointed out that "if Germans reduce their number even by a factor of ten, they would still have over ten times as many as Iceland."

Drugs also are frequently prescribed in combination, with about 70 percent of drugs in Germany being combinations, compared to 30 percent elsewhere. "Germans tend to prescribe combinations of, say, fifteen drugs of which only one is effective," according to Dr. Zoltan Zarday, a Hungarian-born, German-educated internist now practicing in New York. In 1977, for example, one German drug firm was marketing chloramphenicol—an antibiotic with side effects so severe that it is used only very sparingly in many countries—in combination with guaiacol, theophylline (an asthma drug), papaverine, and three vitamins, with a hint that it might be useful in bronchitis and bronchospasm. Another firm was marketing a combination of several B vitamins for use as a painkiller.

Perhaps because both fringe and high-tech medicine are accepted, West Germans are inclined to use all sorts of medicine to an extent that others would regard as excessive. There are more doctors in West Germany per capita than in France, England, or the United States, and the West German patient sees his doctor on the average nearly 12 times a year, compared to 5.2 in France, 5.4 in England, and 4.7 in the United States. West Germans also receive the most prescription items per capita (11.18), compared to 6.53 in the U.K. and 10.04 in France.

All West Germans below a certain income are required to carry health insurance, which is offered by a number of different funds, and unlike the situation in France, where the patient must pay a percentage of medical costs incurred outside the hospital, the German health insurance pays the doctor directly for everything, with no out-of-pocket cost to the patient at all. The German patient therefore has no incentive to economize on medical costs, a situation roughly similar to that found in England. Unlike English doctors, however, the West German doctor has had, until recently, no incentive to economize. German doctors are paid for each act they perform, and they are paid so little for each act (recently, a consultation cost the equivalent of five dollars) that there is a clear incentive to perform as many acts as possible. "The general practitioner is forced to spend extremely little time with each patient. He must earn his money by some technical measure. Every West German doctor has a lot of apparatus in the room—this is the only way to get a higher amount of payment," said Professor Hans Schaefer of the University of Heidelberg. Electrocardiograms, for example, pay three times as much as a consultation.

One study found the average length of consultation to be eighty seconds and another four minutes. Concentrating so many acts in so little time means that the German doctor tends always to be on the run. The British Dr. F. M. Hull baptized the West German GP he observed for a day "The White Rabbit."

Patients seem unlikely to emerge from the doctor's office with the news that they are in good health; and one study showed the Germans had the highest number of diagnoses per capita. An English GP who observed both German hospitals and general practice wrote: "The impression I had that illnesses tended to be spun out as a result of the item-of-service payment system was not contradicted by doctors with whom I spoke."

"Overdoctoring" is a danger here, agreed Dr. Klaus-Dieter Haehn, a professor of family medicine at the University of Hannover. The excesses are particularly apparent with diagnoses and drugs concerning the heart and circulation. Total sales (in German marks) of nitrates, used for angina, in 1981 were 176 million DM in West Germany, compared to 73 million DM in France and 18 million DM in the U.K., countries with roughly similar populations of roughly similar age distributions. When the doses of another type of heart drug, cardiac glycosides (analogs of digitalis), were compared, West Germans used seven times as many doses per capita as did the French and six times as many as the English. Cardiac glycosides are in fact the second most widely prescribed group of drugs in West Germany: only nonnarcotic painkillers are more frequently prescribed. As already mentioned, the rate of heart disease in West Germany seems similar to that in England. The difference seems to lie, rather, in both the concept the Germans have of the heart itself and the way certain cardiac diagnoses are made in Germany.

In the United States, the heart is viewed as a pump, and the major cause of heart pathology is considered to be due to a physical blockage in the plumbing serving the pump. American doctors, therefore, tend to use diagnostic methods (the angiogram) that can show blockage of the pump, and favor treatment methods (the coronary bypass operation) that unblock the tubes. The belief in America that the heart is just a pump is so strong that we became the first nation to seriously think that a machine could in fact replace it.

The Germans knew better, since their concept of the heart is different and, as we are learning little by little, at least in some ways more accurate. For Germans, the heart is not just a pump, but an organ that has a life of its own, one that pulsates in response to a number of different stimuli including the emotions. In other words, the German heart, as opposed to the American heart, retains some of the metaphorical associations with love and the emotions. At first such a concept seems silly, but upon further reflection it offers certain advantages over a purely mechanical model. This way of thinking about the heart probably led Europeans to recognize, long before Americans, that angina pectoris, or lack of oxygen to the heart muscle, can be caused not just by a clogging, but also by a spasm, of the coronary artery, a concept hard to integrate into the mechanical model. Pumps, after all, don't go into spasm. Conversely, while a clogged pipe cannot expand to allow passage, the heart sometimes can. The German cardiologist Dr. Jochen Schaefer, of the

University of Kiel, has pointed out that even a severely clogged artery can often respond by widening, and that the role of heart arrhythmias may be a much more pertinent indicator of the prognosis of heart disease than the morphology of the coronary vascular system.

The German concept of the heart also leads to a difference in certifying heart disease on death certificates. West Germans certify fewer patients as having died of coronary artery disease (clogged arteries), but they certify many more as dying of "other heart disease," undoubtedly reflecting their belief that heart disease is more complex than blocked pipes.

The German way of looking at the heart and what ails it leads to fewer bypass operations and fewer artificial hearts: when the first artificial heart was implanted in West Germany, in fact, the patient wasn't told for two days so as not to disturb him. But the German view also leads to a greater use of drugs for the heart, and the Germans have been in the forefront in developing some of the heart drugs, such as those for arrhythmias and the calcium channel blockers, for the type of spasm that leads to angina.

But another reason for the high use of heart drugs in West Germany is the way many German doctors make a diagnosis known as *Herzinsuffizienz*. In some surveys *Herzinsuffizienz* has accounted for the greatest number of visits to GPs in Germany and the diagnosis has ranked high in other surveys. *Herzinsuffizienz* is usually translated as "congestive heart failure," but while this corresponds to what Germans would probably call severe *Herzinsuffizienz*, what they call early *Herzinsuffizienz* really has no translation into English because it would not be considered a disease in England, France, or America. German doctors often translate it as "cardiac insufficiency," so I have used this term when quoting them directly from statements made in English, but the term is not used very much by English-speaking non-German doctors.

One of the first ways to look for heart disease, of course, is the electrocardiogram. Office-based doctors in West Germany take an ECG in about the same percentage of office visits as doctors in the United States. But since the West German patient sees the doctor roughly three times as often as the U.S patient sees his, the German is nearly three times as likely to have an electrocardiogram in a given year.

The West German doctor also seems more likely to find something wrong with the heart based on the ECG. ECGs are interpretive tests whose results do not necessarily give a clear differentiation between disease and no disease: the area of interpretation as to what is normal and what is not is a wide one. According to Dr. Hans Schaefer, of the University of Heidelberg, a physiologist and doctor with an interest in social medicine, the West German doctor is more likely to find something wrong with an electrocardiogram than is his American counterpart. In a study of the normal population of Hamburg one summer, using German rules of diagnosis, 40 percent of the people were found to have an abnormal ECG. In the same study, using American criteria, Dr. Schaefer said, only 5 percent were found to be abnormal.

But even if the electrocardiogram *is* normal according to German standards, the German doctor may come up with a diagnosis of *Herzinsuffizienz*. One German general practitioner active in medical affairs in the city of Kiel explained that many older people were suffering from *Herzinsuffizienz* even though their electrocardiograms were normal and they were not short of breath (a classic sign of congestive heart failure, although of course it can be a sign of many other things). Any patient, said this doctor, who was about sixty years old and had any *one* of three symptoms—extreme tiredness, urination at night, or edema (waterlogging of tissues)—suffered from *Herzinsuffizienz* and should be given digitalis to prevent further deterioration.

Still other German doctors indicated that digitalis might be prescribed even without the presence of these symptoms. Professor Schadewaldt of Düsseldorf explained that in Germany many doctors consider that a man over sixty has "latent heart insufficiency." Digitalis is used "at the limit of prophylaxis," though as Dr. Schadewaldt explained, "There is no evidence that it can in fact protect the heart before heart insufficiency develops."

According to other observers, West German doctors may begin the "prophylactic" treatment of *Herzinsuffizienz* at even younger ages. "It has been said," wrote William H. Helfand, then president of the pharmaceutical firm Merck Sharp & Dohme's operation in France, "that the German physician considers any heart more than thirty years old to be defective by definition, and he may well prescribe a cardiovascular product for all patients above a certain age."

Dr. Eckart Sturm, editor of the *European Journal of General Practice*, participated in a study of general practitioners in the area of Verden, West Germany, near Hannover, that showed that *Herzinsuffizienz* was the diagnosis accounting for the largest number of visits to the fifteen general practitioners in the study.

While he recognizes that there is a great deal of controversy as to when *Herzinsuffizienz* should be treated, Dr. Sturm firmly believed that the disease should be diagnosed and treated in its "earliest" stages—that is, when the symptoms are slight. "We see the fourth stage of cardiac insufficiency very seldom," he said. "This is because we give digitalis very soon, sooner than would be done in the United States. If the heart cannot pump, it does not get enough blood itself, and it deteriorates further."

Why, then, do the English and Americans not treat cardiac insufficiency at this early stage?

Part of the explanation, Dr. Sturm said, was that the English and Americans typically use twice the dose of digitalis used in Germany. When younger German doctors tried to use English doses, he explained, they ended up with a 20 percent complication rate.

An additional reason Americans tend not to treat the early stages of *Herzinsuffizienz*, he said, concerns another drug used to treat the condition, strophanthin. This German drug was marketed in two doses, one twice that of the other. Only the higher dose was sold in the United States, said Dr. Sturm, resulting in a high complication rate including heart attacks. But what evidence does he have that giving digitalis prevents the later stages of *Herzinsuffizienz?* Dr. Sturm answered that a famous German doctor, Professor Reindell of Freiberg, had said this over twenty years ago.

Another participant in the Verden study, Dr. Klaus-Dieter Haehn, of the University of Hannover Medical School, had a relatively low rate of visits by patients with *Herzinsuffizienz* although the rate would still be considered high by English and American standards. When asked about the frequent use of digitalis, Dr. Haehn admitted, "Nobody knows whether it is good or bad. We had a meeting with cardiologists on this question, and they weren't much help. They made two suggestions: one, that we could use cardiac catheterization to make the diagnosis, which the patients wouldn't like; or two, we could make a trial of digitalis for four weeks. The problem with this is that you really cannot stop if the patient says he feels better."

Dr. Haehn nevertheless attempted to find out exactly what digitalis was doing for his patients. He selected eighty who were receiving the drug: twenty he decided to keep on the drug because they had objective signs of heart failure, and he suggested to the other sixty that they stop. Forty did. "They are still alive," Dr. Haehn said with a smile, admitting that some wanted to go back on the drug. "I have four hundred patients with the diagnosis of cardiac insufficiency," he said. "If I could take three-quarters of them off digitalis, it would be a great saving for the social insurance system."

Non-German doctors familiar with the German habit of prescribing small doses of digitalis tend to regard the practice as a harmless use of placebos. "Digitalis is used here as a general tonic," explained the British Dr. Mark Ball, who practices in Hannover, "something we were warned against doing in medical school." The practice, he observed, is apparently an old tradition.

"A lot of German cardiac preparations contain digitalis," said Dr. R. S. Inch, senior vice president of the Sterling-Europa drug company, based in Paris. "It's not all that silly. The British went through a phase when they gave digitalis until a person was 'digitalized' or on the verge of being poisoned," said Dr. Inch, who is British. "There was a tendency for doctors on the Continent to give small doses, which seldom produced side effects and were probably beneficial."

But do small doses of digitalis really have a tonic effect? "I don't know, but I'm sure they have," said Dr. Inch. "An awful lot cannot be proven, but if the patient feels better . . ."

All countries have their "wastebasket diagnosis," that is, what the doctor calls vague symptoms that cannot be ascribed to anything else; but what causes West Germans to ascribe everything to their heart? Dr. Willibald Nagler, physiatrist-in-chief at New York Hospital–Cornell Medical Center, noted that "In Austria and Germany there are two or three diagnoses that everybody gets at age sixty—*Herzinsuffizienz*, gastritis, and gallbladder dyskinesia." Dr. Nagler, of Austrian origin himself, suggested that taking digitalis for *Herzinsuffizienz* is something of a status symbol. "When you're a fashionable old gentleman in Austria, it doesn't hurt your standing to take heart medicine. Here in the United States a patient would probably deny taking medicine. There, it shows his status."

Regina Molders-Kober, a medical sociologist working at the medical school in Hannover, suggested that it might be partly a linguistic problem. In German, she explained, there is no word for "chest pain," only words for "breast pain" and "heart pain." In fact, heart pain was the seventh most common reason for contact with general practitioners in one study with West German general practitioners.

Dr. Zarday suggested the concern with the heart and the particular form it took in West Germany was a heritage of romanticism, particularly the large number of German romantic literary figures with something wrong with their "hearts." And Professor Moos related the diagnosis to the German character: "I continue to like the term *Herzinsuffizienz* because it says a great deal about Germans and their various ills."

The influence of German romanticism was evoked by another doctor, Herbert Viefhues, who holds the chair of social medicine at the University of Bochum. He offered romanticism as an explanation for another group of peculiarly German diagnoses: low blood pressure, circulatory collapse, and vasovegetative dystonia.

All these diagnoses relate to the circulation (the German word is *Kreislauf*), and there can be no question that Germans are inordinately concerned about theirs. Besides the large number of diagnoses of and treatments for impaired circulation, poor circulation is held in West Germany to be the underlying cause of many diseases of specific organs.

Low blood pressure, for example, is referred to by the English as the "German disease" because of the German concern for and many ways of treating a blood pressure that is lower than normal. The second most common reason given by West Germans for physician visits is vertigo-dizziness (preceded only by cough in the number-one spot), which is often taken to indicate low blood pressure, a condition not even mentioned in a similar U.S. survey. According to Owen L. Wade, dean of the faculty of medicine and dentistry, University of Birmingham, England, in a recent year the frequency of consultation for low blood pressure was 0 per million persons in England and 163 per million in Germany. And in a recent *Rote Liste*, the German catalog of available prescription drugs, no fewer than eighty-five drugs were listed for the treatment of low blood pressure.

While low blood pressure was occasionally mentioned in U.S. medical literature in the post–World War II era, it apparently failed to catch the popular imagination and waned in the 1950s to the point where it is now considered a nondisease and indeed a contributor to longevity. The one case where hypotension would be treated is a rare condition known as orthostatic hypotension, which sometimes causes patients to faint upon arising.

"Hypotension [low blood pressure] is a German diagnosis," explained Dr. Jack Froom, professor of family medicine at the

SUNY Health Science Center at Stony Brook, New York, who is working with an international group trying to standardize diagnostic terms used in general practice. "This would not be a disease in the United States. It is, in fact, associated with long life. We would perhaps treat a patient if his blood pressure were so low he fainted, but Germans consider a low reading, with no symptoms, as something to be treated. Many women have eighty as their upper reading. The Germans could not tolerate this, whereas we think it's all to the better."

"The diagnosis of low blood pressure makes American doctors laugh," said Dr. Inch. "Americans think it is almost malpractice to treat low blood pressure."

"In England," said Dr. Ball, "we are taught that low blood pressure may be unpleasant, but we should be happy to have it."

The statement that low blood pressure is unpleasant also produced disagreement: doctors I talked to in West Germany believe that hypotension causes tiredness, while most doctors elsewhere believe otherwise. Dr. Geoffrey Rose, professor of epidemiology at the London School of Hygiene and Tropical Medicine, emphatically denied that low blood pressure causes tiredness. Several studies have shown, he said, that people develop symptoms of tiredness only *after* they are told their blood pressure is low. Whether German fatigue is the same as English fatigue may, of course, be open to question.

German doctors nevertheless persist: "I think low blood pressure will be of interest in industrial medicine because people will be tired with it," said Professor Schadewaldt, who explained that low blood pressure was very common in the starvation period following World War II but had decreased enormously in recent years, since the best cure is good eating.

Professor Hans Schaefer of Heidelberg explained: "If a patient is tired, you give a drug that raises the blood pressure. They take one pill and everything is okay. I myself have low blood pressure, and when I take one pill, everything is fine." The pills given in Germany often contain a mixture of adrenaline, which raises the blood pressure, and sugar, which concurrently raises the blood sugar.

Perhaps because it is sometimes a manifestation of low blood pressure, or perhaps because it fits in so well with the German emphasis on suppressed emotion, a faint is taken more seriously in West Germany than it would be in England or America. "When I first came to Germany," said Dr. Ball, "I tried to understand why people were getting so worked up with a faint." He explained that such concerns were important to him as a psychiatrist because he often had cause to prescribe drugs where fainting was a reasonably common side effect.

Dr. Ball also said he was mystified by the German concern over their circulation in general: "I didn't know what people meant when they talked about having trouble with their circulation. I would have thought claudication or cold hands, but this wasn't the case."

Poor circulation, in fact, is blamed for a broad spectrum of complaints in West Germany, from tired legs and varicose veins to *Kreislaufkollaps*, or circulatory collapse, which itself can range from fainting to heart attack. The actor Kurt Raab, writing about the death of Rainer Werner Fassbinder, described the cause as a combination of stimulant drugs and depressant sleeping pills that "brought the severely strained circulation to collapsing submission"; an American writing about the same topic would undoubtedly have written less poetically that Fassbinder died of a drug overdose. Since circulation affects all organs of the body, underlying poor circulation can be held responsible for almost any illness and indeed in West Germany it often is.

Why such concern over the circulation in West Germany? One common response is that Germans tend to be fat and therefore do have poorer circulation. Another is that such beliefs are created by the pharmaceutical industry to sell products. But the British Dr. Dukes believes that while the pharmaceutical industry is indeed good at exploiting such beliefs, drug companies do not invent concern about the circulation out of thin air. "You cannot get Dutchmen and Englishmen to worry about their venous circulation," he observed.

A non-German doctor suggested that there might be lots of money in diagnosing diseases of the circulation, but Professor Viefhues of Bochum rejected this explanation. "If the German doctor were after money, he would diagnose liver problems rather than circulatory problems," he said, having just been informed about the French tendency to blame many things on the liver. "The liver business would be well paid—you could do twelve or sixteen analyses." Rather, explained Dr. Viefhues, the concern with the circulation stems from the central European cultural perspective on physiology. "There is a basic assumption of equilibrium or balance—that antagonistic forces should be kept in balance."

This idea of balance means that blood pressure should be controlled by a balance between adrenaline output and adrenaline antagonists, he said, and that there is a balance between the heart and the peripheral circulation, with the peripheral circulation being an autonomously acting organ. "A massive amount of blood can sink in your peripheral circulation," he said, noting that he thought that U.S. research was too focused on the heart and German research perhaps too much on the peripheral circulation.

Dr. Viefhues also mentioned Rudolf Virchow, perhaps the most influential doctor in Germany to this day, as having something to do with German ideas about circulation. While Virchow, who lived in the nineteenth century, was not considered part of the German movement of romantic medicine, and in fact rebelled against it, his biographer notes that Virchow was nevertheless influenced by the movement. Virchow felt that many diseases, such as dyspepsia, muscle spasms, and hyperesthesia, were due to a lack of venous circulation. He also explained gastric ulcer as not merely a result of hyperacidity but of a concomitant local circulatory disturbance of the mucosa of the stomach. Such diseases, he felt, could be cured by correcting the circulatory disturbance, thereby providing blood to the tissues.

One popular way to treat complaints felt to be due to bad circulation is hydrotherapy, or water therapy, and one that several West German doctors recommended to me was Kneipp therapy, which in its alternation of hot and cold showers fits in perfectly with German romantic ideas of polarity and balance. This particular form of hydrotherapy owes its origins to a nineteenth-century preacher named Sebastian Kneipp. The therapy usually consists, Dr. Sturm explained, of a shower of one minute of warm water, followed by a shower of twenty seconds of cold water, then another one minute of warm water followed by another twenty seconds of cold water.

Dr. Sturm explained that he uses hydrotherapy on himself daily as a preventive measure, as do members of his family. "You do a different part each day," he explained. "Today I did my scalp. I will do my back tomorrow and my stomach the day after. If you are using hydrotherapy to actually treat a disease rather than as a preventive measure, then you may use more water on the diseased part, for example, the liver or the neck." A 1980 book on Kneipp therapy used by West German doctors recommends as therapy for a patient with low blood pressure to have, on Mondays, an early bath of the upper body, a morning knee shower alternating between hot and cold water, an afternoon arm shower, and a walk in fifteen inches of water (known in Germany as "Kneipping") in the evening; on Tuesdays, an early bath of the lower body, an arm bath with rosemary in the morning, an alternating hot and cold footbath in the afternoon, and Kneipping in the evening, and so on for the rest of the week, except Sunday.

Professor Schaefer of Heidelberg claimed that one Kneipp treatment, putting cold water on the knee, "makes another man or woman of you. You cannot cure insufficiency of the heart muscle, but it is wonderful for a hangover."

Even the British Dr. Ball believed in Kneipp. "Kneipp is not really fringe," he said, when I brought up the name in a discussion we were having about fringe medicine in Germany. "They can prove it works. I once got rid of chilblains [a mild form of frostbite common in England because of the lack of central heating] that way myself."

While Kneipp therapy can be taken anywhere that hot and cold water is available, there is a special Kneipp spa at Bad Wörishofen, a sleepy little town in southern Germany where West Germans go to devote themselves to Kneipp therapy. After so many doctors had told me about Kneipp, I decided to visit Bad Wörishofen myself. I found there a Kneipp monument, a Kneipp museum, a Kneippianum (a building in which Kneipp therapy is given), and a Kneipp Street, where people buy Kneipp sandals and eat Kneipp rolls. One of the main activities in Bad Wörishofen is, of course, Kneipping, and public pools are maintained in the parks for that purpose.

The idea of balance was also invoked to explain yet another German diagnosis, vasovegetative dystonia. Literally, vasovegetative dystonia is supposed to be an imbalance of the autonomic nervous system, with the parasympathetic system predominating over the sympathetic system. It is characterized by heart palpitations, arrhythmias, sweating, lack of appetite, bad sleep, and trembling. In English this diagnosis is called autonomic dysautotonia, but practically no one uses the term. Dr. Schadewaldt said that in West Germany, "Younger doctors recognize it as a psychosomatic disease—older ones treat it as a somatic disease, sometimes with rye ergot [a drug often used for migraine headaches]." Dr. Schadewaldt, who was a prisoner of war in Strasbourg, said it corresponded in large part to the French diagnosis of spasmophilia.

"When confronted with a patient, the German doctor has a paradigm, or model, of the sympathetic and parasympathetic nervous system," said Dr. Henk Lamberts, a Dutch general practitioner from Rotterdam. "He fits the patient into this system and then finds a therapy for it."

"It's one of those polite diagnoses," said Dr. Ball with a laugh (Germans have a special word—*Verlegenheitsdiagnostik*—for "polite diagnosis"). "In England, it is immediately recognized as being psychogenic. It is a diagnosis you can make without offending the patient."

"I had forgotten about that diagnosis," said Dr. Nagler of New York Hospital. "Germans like romantic, nondescriptive types of diagnosis."

"Vasovegetative dystonia is a necessary diagnosis because patients do not want to be thought of as crazy," said the sociologist Mrs. Molders-Kober.

"We need this diagnosis for patients without organic signs," said Dr. Haehn. "These patients have problems with their lives, and treatment is very difficult—it depends on the patient. Some you treat with psychological methods. You can suggest autogenous training, or put them into groups. For some you give Valium. However, you cannot generally give psychotherapy to older persons, or to simple people."

The legacy of Virchow may also help to explain another peculiarity of present-day West German medicine: their comparatively low use of antibiotics. Virchow is probably best known outside West Germany for his elaboration of the theory of cellular pathology, which was riddled with Virchow's democratic political leanings. Just as German political philosophers of the nineteenth century, such as Hegel, compared city-states to cells, scientists such as Virchow compared cells to city-states. According to his biographer, Erwin H. Ackerknecht, Virchow recognized that cells were both dependent and independent but emphasized the latter largely for politico-philosophical reasons. Virchow saw the body as a cell-state, with disease being merely a conflict of the citizens of that state provoked by external forces. Like the French who stress the importance of *terrain*, he deemphasized external causes of disease, focusing instead upon disease as altered (read: "imbalanced") physiology. When Virchow was sent to investigate an outbreak of typhus in Upper Silesia, he came back with a report that people wouldn't have caught the typhus had they been living in a democratic political system (presumably because their living conditions would have been better). Virchow also resisted the evidence of the Hungarian physician Ignaz Semmelweis and of Oliver Wendell Holmes that childbed fever was caused by germs. He argued that while germs might be a necessary cause of disease, they were not a sufficient cause; i.e., something else—for example, a lowered resistance—had to be present for the patient to become ill.

That West German doctors still pay less attention to the germ and greater attention to the patient's resistance, is apparent both from drug utilization statistics and from talking with West German doctors. Not one group of antibiotics made the top twenty types of prescription drugs in Germany in the 1984 British Office of Health Economics Report, and another comparison showed that the use of systemic antibiotics in Germany was less than half that of France and also considerably less than that in Great Britain, both of which consume relatively fewer antibiotics than we do in the United States.

"We never give antibiotics for a common cold, as I've heard is done in England and America," said the same doctor who prescribed digitalis for tired patients. "On the first visit we would only give aspirin. After five days we would do a blood sedimentation and listen to the lungs. Then we might give antibiotics."

"We consider that the body can get rid of a fever on its own," said Dr. Gisela Brandt, a resident in family practice at the University Medical School in Hannover.

"A lot of people have an exaggerated fear of penicillin here, and a doctor is considered bad if he gives penicillin too soon," said Dr. Ball.

"There are no real indications for giving antibiotics in private practice," said Dr. Peter Naumann, a professor of infectious diseases at the University of Düsseldorf. "If a patient needs an antibiotic, he generally needs to be in the hospital."

Dr. Naumann went on: "The German patient will say, 'I am severely sick; I must take penicillin.' "

Just finding a bacteria associated with a disease, Dr. Naumann said, doesn't mean that the bacteria has caused the symptoms. He explained that the medical microbiologists in West Germany are trained to evaluate whether the microbes found in association with disease are causative or not. They would give antibiotics only if the microbes were causative.

Dr. Naumann, as well as his colleague, Dr. Harry Rosin, pointed out that even before the era of antibiotics few patients with bacterial infections died, and most would not die now.

But would the patients get better more quickly with antibiotics? The West German patient doesn't have to worry about getting well more quickly because his illness is paid for by health and other forms of social insurance, Dr. Rosin responded, perhaps a good illustration of another of Virchow's statements, that "medicine is a social science, and politics is only medicine on a grand scale."

While there may be some disadvantages to the patient in such restrictive use of antibiotics, there are two important advantages. One, of course, is that antibiotics, like other drugs, are associated with side effects that can be worse than the original disease. The other is that widespread antibiotic use leads to the development of antibiotic-resistant bacteria that have caused a number of serious infections. According to Dr. Naumann, such outbreaks of antibiotic-resistant germs have been less of a problem in West Germany than in many other countries, particularly in hospitals such as his own where antibiotics are used very parsimoniously.

The relative importance given by German medicine to "inner" causes as compared to outer ones is seen in other areas of German medicine as well. While the French are responsible for the original division of pathology into "inner" and "outer," it was the Germans who elevated the specialty of *Innere Medizin*— which became the less mystical and more mechanical "internal medicine" in English—to its present-day power in West Germany and the United States.

German psychiatry has also traditionally considered inner causes more important than environmental ones in mental disease. According to J. Marshall Townsend, an anthropologist at Syracuse University who compared attitudes toward mental illness of both psychiatrists and their patients in West Germany and the United States, "Generally speaking, contemporary German psychiatry dichotomizes between 'sick' and 'healthy': it attributes more behavioral traits to biological causes than does American psychiatry, and it therefore presumes that 'personality' is a less labile and malleable entity. Apparently, Germans tend to view mental disorders as endogenous in origin, relatively incurable, and less subject to environmental influence than do Americans."

Dr. Townsend found the German patients generally agreed with their doctors that mental illness is a biological and virtually incurable phenomenon. For the American patients in his study, on the other hand, "mental illness" resided in behavioral deviance rather than in an innate, organic condition. Both mental-health professionals and laymen in America emphasized that "to maintain good health, a person must 'try' to get well, he should avoid worry, learn good emotional habits, and read books on peace of mind."

At least part of the generally pessimistic German view of mental illness is attributed to the German psychiatrist Emil Kraepelin, who lived from 1856 to 1926 and whose classification of psychiatric disease was mentioned in the chapter on French medicine. Kraepelin was the first to distinguish between dementia praecox, what is now considered schizophrenia, and manic-depressive psychosis. Kraepelin's choice of the term *dementia*, which implies incurability, was felt to be the nihilistic hallmark of a reactionary psychiatry that reflected the intellectual climate of the Germany of Emperor Wilhelm II.

This pessimism concerning the curability of mental illness persisted well into the twentieth century, and may have eased the way for the Nazi regime to have more than 100,000 mentally ill persons killed as "life not worth living" until the practice was stopped in 1941 due to pressure from the German public.

The psychiatric profession in Germany has never really recovered from the reputation it earned for its role in these killings during the war.

"It's not really respectable to be a psychiatrist here," said Dr. Ball. "To call yourself a psychiatrist is a disaster." Were he to establish a private practice, Dr. Ball said, he might consider calling himself a psychotherapist.

"A psychiatrist was always considered a queer man handling queer persons," said Dr. Viefhues.

Most psychiatrists in Germany are neuropsychiatrists, with training in both neurology and psychiatry. "People can therefore go to a neuropsychiatrist without it being obvious that they are seeing a psychiatrist," said Dr. Ball.

The unacceptability of psychiatry may account for the fact that the diagnosis of neurosis is very uncommon in West German general practice compared to other countries. While neurosis was the leading diagnosis made by general practitioners in England in the Office of Health Economics study, more commonly made than hypertension or arthritis and accounting for 5 percent of total diagnoses, and the second most common diagnosis in France, accounting for 4.1 percent, with an additional 2.5 percent of diagnoses being for nervousness and debility, neuroses did not make the top twenty diagnoses in West Germany, meaning that fewer than 1 percent of German diagnoses were neuroses. The nearest diagnosis was physical disorders of psychic origin (what we would call psychosomatic, or psychogenic), accounting for 2.2 percent of total diagnoses. West Germany also has a somewhat lower use of psychoactive drugs than either England or France.

Still another legacy of romanticism to German medicine is the healing powers accorded to nature, whether it be in the form of long walks in the forests, mud baths, or herbal medicine.

The medical use of spas is even more widespread than in France, and plants are more widely used for their healing powers. Of 8,250 preparations listed in the German pharmacopoeia the *Rote Liste*, 1,400 were of herbal base.

About one-fifth of German M.D.'s practice either homeopathy or anthroposophic medicine, as well as *Phytotherapie*, or plant therapy. These forms of therapy are recognized under the West German health system, and have to some extent been upgraded following World War II. Under recent German drug laws, the alternative medicines will have to be shown to be harmless, but there is no requirement that they be shown to be effective, and their continued use will be decided by commissions composed of practitioners of the particular alternative therapies (the usefulness of anthroposophic medicine, for example, will be decided by doctors certified in anthroposophic medicine).

The anthroposophic system is based on the philosophic system of Rudolf Steiner, a worldview that, according to Paul Unschuld of Johns Hopkins University, is shared by a significant proportion of the West German population. Steiner, like many German philosophers, rejected the purely empirical view that the world of the senses is the primary reality: rather, he believed, knowledge of the spiritual world was something to be grasped in the same way a geometrical concept is grasped. A true romantic, he felt that feelings are organs of perception just like eyes and ears.

In 1919, Steiner extended his ideas to medicine, in a scheme that contains many of the balance and polarity concepts that characterize romanticism. Disease was attributed to an imbalance between the nerve-sense or "cold" pole and the metabolic "hot" pole. Overactivity of the former was responsible for degenerative conditions and tumors, and overactivity of the latter caused inflammation. Perhaps not surprisingly, the cold and warm streams come together in the heart.

Steiner gave many indications for the preparation of specific remedies, but their activities were not to be understood primarily in terms of the chemistry of their active ingredients. Today, two anthroposophical pharmaceutical firms manufacture the remedies. Perhaps the best known is Iscador, which is made from mistletoe and used to treat cancer by stimulating the immune response of the body. Two large anthroposophical hospitals were opened in West Germany in the 1970s, and there are at least ten smaller hospitals practicing anthroposophical medicine, staffed with doctors who have received mainstream medical training in West Germany as well as their additional training in anthroposophic medicine.

Steiner's system also uses many of the concepts of homeopathy developed earlier by the German doctor Samuel Christian Hahnemann. Homeopathy differs from allopathy (Hahnemann's name for mainstream medicine) in several ways. While allopathic medicine often prescribes a medicine designed to suppress a symptom—for example, aspirin to bring down a fever—homeopathy prescribes a medicine that would produce the symptoms of the disease in a healthy person. Malaria, for example, produces fever, and quinine, when given to a healthy person, also produces fever—yet quinine alleviates the symptoms of malaria, including fever. From this observation, Hahnemann formulated the principle that "like is healed by like." Another difference between the two approaches is that individual *terrains* are considered much more important in homeopathic medicine than in allopathic medicine. Still a third distinguishing principle is that, in contrast to allopathic medicine, where larger doses are considered to be stronger, in homeopathy the most dilute dose is considered to be the most effective. The homeopathic remedies considered the strongest are in fact so dilute that they probably do not even contain one molecule of the so-called effective substance; the effectiveness of the medication is judged to be due to vibrations in the water induced by being shaken with the substance in question.

Most American doctors would say that if homeopathy works, it must be via the placebo effect; and the more liberal among them might concede that homeopathy is useful as a placebo and at least does no harm. But European homeopaths believe that their medicine works beyond the placebo effect: homeopathic remedies are used in veterinary medicine, where it is difficult to conceive of placebos being effective, and a few randomized clinical trials have even shown homeopathic remedies to be more effective than placebo.

Exactly how contact with homeopathy can influence the thinking of nonhomeopathic doctors was brought home to me in the summer of 1985. In the course of covering a meeting in New York on digestive diseases, I came upon the poster presentation of a German professor of internal medicine who had discovered that a larger concentration of alcohol is less irritating to the stomach than a more dilute concentration and that cognac and whiskey were less irritating than wine and beer. After asking the professor a few questions for my article, I remarked that his results seemed to validate to some extent homeopathic beliefs. He just smiled.

Later that day, when at the end of a long session I took a drink at the hotel bar, I struck up a conversation with a surgeon from Washington, D.C., who was also attending the meeting. Over my cognac, I tried to explain the German professor's findings. The American surgeon found them impossible to believe and said that he would have repeated the experiments and in no case would have published such results, since they were obviously wrong. I also talked with a fellow journalist who thought the experiments were weak because there weren't enough patients, although American medical journalism is replete with reports of viruses being found in single patients with a given disease.

It proved a good lesson in how our expectations and culture values influence how we view even the results of experience. For while some German practices seem strange, considering alternative ways of looking at the body can open our eyes to new insights and discoveries. Perhaps larger doses are *not* always stronger doses, and indeed the recent concept that some drugs have therapeutic windows—points at which increasing the dose results in lessened effectiveness—partially corroborates some aspects of homeopathic theory if not all its practices. Had we Americans a less mechanical view of the human heart, we might have accepted earlier the idea that angina can be caused by spasm, that coronary artery surgery is not always the answer to heart problems, and that a mechanical heart would not have the same ability to adjust to the strains of the environment that an organic heart has. If we held some of the German ideas of balance, we might be less likely to recommend extremes of treatment that eventually turn out to be harmful. If we had paid more attention to the healing compounds found in plants, we might have a wider variety of effective drugs today. And if we used antibiotics more as the West Germans do, these important drugs might be more effective when we really need them.

Great Britain:
Economy, Empiricism, and Keeping the Upper Lip Stiff

JACK: Oh, before the end of the week I shall have got rid of him. I'll say he died in Paris of apoplexy. Lots of people die of apoplexy, quite suddenly, don't they?
ALGERNON: Yes, but it's hereditary, my dear fellow. It's the sort of thing that runs in families. You had much better say a severe chill.
—Oscar Wilde
The Importance of Being Earnest

My wife has two topics of conversation: the royal family and her bowels.
—From the movie
A Private Function

At the Strasbourg meeting on breast cancer, one of the British surgeons present pointed out that the lumpectomy would tend to be favored by British surgeons for a reason other than its aesthetic results: it's an easier operation. While an American or French surgeon gets more money for more difficult operations, and would therefore be better paid for performing a radical mastectomy than a lumpectomy, the British surgeon receives the same salary no matter how he treats the disease.

The most striking characteristic of British medicine is its economy. The British do less of nearly everything. While British patients see the doctor slightly more often (5.4 visits a year) than the American (4.7) or French (5.2) patient, their visits last only about six minutes, compared to 15 to 20 minutes in France and America. The British doctor is much less likely to do routine examinations than his colleagues in France or America. One study showed only three such exams among a group of British GPs compared to 188 among a similar number of Iowa GPs. British doctors take the blood pressure, throat swabs, and temperature much less often than do doctors in other European countries and North America. "I've watched the English do examinations, and they do minimal investigations and examinations," said Dr. Jack Froom, of the department of family medicine at the State University of New York (SUNY) at Stony Brook. "When I was watching in England, a kid came in with an earache and the doctor looked at *that* ear. Here, we would at least have the patient undress to the waist, particularly with a child because it's so easy to undress a child, and would have looked at the throat and lungs. The information would probably make no difference, but our reflexes are different."

The British patient receives half the number of X rays as the American and each X ray will use half the film. If widespread spots are found on this chest X ray, British textbooks will give 85 causes for them, compared to 125 causes given by American textbooks.

British doctors prescribe fewer drugs (6.53 per capita) than French (10.04) or West German (11.18) doctors. They are unlikely to use calcium supplements, lactobacillus, or the kinds of peripheral vasodilators used in France at all, and they use fewer heart drugs than the French and Germans, and fewer anticancer drugs than the Americans. The British patient is half as likely to have surgery of any kind as an American and one-sixth as likely to undergo coronary bypass. Should the doctor decide that surgery is necessary, the surgery itself will probably be less extensive: there will be no lymph node dissection for testicular cancer, for example, which Professor Michael Baum of King's College Hospital referred to as "an antique, barbarous custom."

High-technology medicine such as renal dialysis, CAT scanners, and intensive-care beds are much less in evidence than elsewhere. When the Wellcome Museum of the History of Medicine in London set up a display on coronary care units, the skin of the mannequin representing the patient was deliberately made dark enough to imply that this was the sort of medical care reserved for Middle Eastern oil sheikhs who came to use private doctors, not the sort English patients could expect on the National Health Service.

Even vitamin requirements are smaller. The recommended daily allowance for vitamin C is half that of most other countries, including the United States, and the recommended value for calcium is 500 milligrams, as compared to 800 milligrams in the U.S. "On the whole the British recommendations tend to be careful or prudent rather than generous," said one British nutritionist. And until the dose of glucose to be used for glucose tolerance tests was standardized a few years ago at 75 grams, the British used 50 grams compared to the American 100 grams.

Very few screening exams are done, and when they are, they are done less often than in other countries. While it is now recognized in Britain that screening for high blood pressure is important, the recommendation is that an adult should have his blood pressure taken once every five years. Similarly, the doctor is paid extra for doing Pap smears, but only for women over thirty-five and only once every five years.

As a consequence, the British patient is less likely to be labeled as sick by his doctor: you can't be diagnosed as having hypertension if nobody ever takes your blood pressure. But even when blood pressure is taken, the British have a higher threshold for disease. "Some people here [in the United States] believe that a diastolic pressure over ninety should be treated," said Dr. Thomas Pickering of New York Hospital–Cornell Medical Center. "In England, they would probably not treat unless it was over one hundred." In a comparison with Dutch GPs, British doctors diagnosed only half as many patients as being hypertensive or having urinary tract infections, and only one-fifth as

many as being obese. "Dutch doctors are more likely to look
for obesity in their patients and to label it as a 'disease' whereas
there may well be more tolerance of obesity by British doctors,"
concluded the authors of the comparison. British psychiatrists
are also more likely to pronounce a patient mentally well, or
at least not as sick, as their colleagues in other countries. British
psychiatrists noticed fewer symptoms than did their French
counterparts in a three-way comparison, and, in another study,
noticed only half as many symptoms as did American psychiatrists. Concerning a well-publicized American study where eight
men posing as schizophrenics were not recognized as sane by
the staffs of mental hospitals, one British psychiatrist responded
that the pose of schizophrenia wouldn't have been sufficient to
get the men admitted to a British mental hospital. If a man
"presented to a British mental hospital complaining only of a
single auditory hallucination, he might well be advised to go
home like a good man, get a decent night's rest, and come back
in the morning."

The usual American interpretation of British economy in
medicine is that the British have had a Draconian rationing
placed upon them by the National Health Service. The emphasis
on doing as little as possible, they argue, is only a rationalization
for cutbacks in services due mainly to lack of funds.

Certainly, there is a degree of rationing, which is particularly
evident in the purchase of high technology and in hospital beds
for elective surgery. There is also rationing in the number of
specialists. There are no "specialoids"—a term coined by Dr.
John Fry when he was in the United States ("I thought it nicer
than pseudospecialists")—such as internists and pediatricians
who actually act largely as general practitioners despite their
extra training. There are half as many surgeons per capita as in
the United States (and in England, unlike the United States,
only specialist surgeons are allowed to operate), and only slightly
over one hundred cardiologists in all of the health service. Dr.
Osler Peterson of the University of Pennsylvania explained how
this might raise the threshold for an individual operation: "I've

heard U.S. surgeons say that if a man has to get up once a night to urinate, this is not an excuse for prostatectomy. If he has to get up twice, then prostatectomy is indicated, because getting up twice in the night will disturb sleep. In England, the surgeon would be likely to say prostatectomy is indicated if a man has to urinate three times in the night, since they have fewer surgeons to do it."

But not all the English economies can be explained by direct rationing. Sir Raymond Hoffenberg, of the Royal College of Physicians in London, could think of only two instances where physicians' liberties to prescribe what they thought best were limited on a national level: in the late 1960s when a ban was placed on heart transplants (following a public outcry that heart transplants were experimental and shouldn't be used yet on patients) and in 1984 when a law passed to cut down on the use of psychotropic drugs made certain drugs unobtainable on the National Health Service. English GPs, who handle the bulk of all medical complaints, have had fewer restrictions as to which tests or medications they could prescribe than their colleagues in France, West Germany, or even the United States. Yet British doctors prescribe half as much medicine as their colleagues in France and West Germany and, at least according to one study, one-eighth the number of lab tests as do Canadian doctors.

One explanation for British medical economy lies in the incentive system for doctors built into the National Health Service. All patients must be registered with a general practitioner, who alone decides whether they should be seen by a specialist. General practitioners are paid in three ways: by a "capitation" (per capita) fee for each patient on their list (with more for patients over sixty-five and over seventy-five), by a small salary, and by fee-for-service for various preventive items that the National Health Service believes should be encouraged, such as immunizations. Approximately half the GP's income comes from capitation fees, so the main way the British GP can increase his income is by getting as many patients on his list as possible, preferably patients who rarely have to see the doctor. "A patient with asthma would be a liability in England," said Dr. David Winstanley, a pathologist. "The ideal patient in England is one like myself who hasn't seen a doctor since 1969," he said in 1981.

Specialists are salaried, so the only way they can increase *their* income is to receive a merit award. Taking private patients is an option, but in spite of all the publicity given to private medicine in Britain, less than 10 percent of the population resorts to it.

So in contrast to other countries, where GPs and specialists often fight over patients, and where general surgeons and gynecologists fight over who should be treating breast cancer, specialists in Britain do not fight over patients, at least not sick ones. In fact some specialists tend to define their specialties as narrowly as possible to keep their workload down. More patients do not mean more money, and they can only cut down on civilized institutions such as the tea break. Surgeons don't like to get "GP rubbish" such as minor surgery, and in most parts of Britain the neurosurgeon accepts less than 5 percent of patients admitted to the hospital with head injuries, while spinal and peripheral nerve trauma are dealt with almost exclusively by orthopedic surgeons. "My father was an endocrinologist," said one English doctor, "and only in private practice would he see 'endocrine rubbish' such as obesity."

This system, in which the danger of "underdoctoring" is greater than the danger of "overdoctoring," was not suddenly imposed on the British medical profession against their wishes but indeed grew out of the existing one. Capitation was used in the nineteenth century by societies of miners known as friendly societies, which, according to Brian Abel-Smith, professor of social administration at the University of London, were very cost-conscious and often criticized doctors who they felt were prescribing too much. Many specialists didn't get paid at all for their hospital work, which they did as charity. When the National Health Service was started in 1911, a time when, Dr.

Peterson pointed out, "there was still land to be homesteaded in the United States," both capitation and salary were well established as ways of paying the doctor. The NHS was extended to the entire population in the aftermath of World War II.

"I started practicing one year before the NHS took effect in 1948," said Dr. Fry, a GP who is author of numerous books about general practice around the globe. "Nothing changed very much except we didn't have to send out monthly bills, and didn't have 20 percent bad debts. We even use the same envelopes for record keeping used before 1948," he said, showing one of the approximately four-by-six envelopes. "It was just after the war, when money was scarce, and if they had changed the files NHS would have been faced with the expense of new ones and doctors would have had to buy new filing cabinets. The small files teach us not to write down too much."

"The British health service," said Dr. Fry, "is based in the conservative, critical questioning and cynicism of doctors. Our training is very much bedside training and treatment. It's highly self-critical. You are taught to question the need for things being done. You are trained to think what is really necessary, why do you do it, what the results are. Does modern medical technology do any good? Is it better than not doing anything?"

"In Britain," said nutritionist Dr. Anthony Leeds, when asked about vitamin requirements, "medical people tend to be conservatives, cautious about doing things generally."

"Most British doctors are within a certain range of orthodoxy," said Dr. Winstanley. "Many of the fringe practitioners in the West End of London are Eastern European. The brainwashing we are subjected to in British medical school discourages this." The one fringe medicine that does have a certain following is, interestingly enough, homeopathy, which might appeal to the British sense of economy because of the small doses used. It also helps that the Royal Family uses homeopathic doctors and remedies.

The medical school training in turn reflects several aspects of British society. By far the strongest philosophical movement in Britain has been that of the empiricists Locke, Berkeley, and Hume. For empiricists, all knowledge comes from experience, not theory or thought. In contrast to Descartes's plan of evolving the universe from a thought, the British philosopher Francis Bacon urged society to try evolving thought from the universe.

The whole of British law as well as government reflects this type of thinking. While on the Continent legal codes have been drawn up that anticipate disputes, in Britain law is based on the interpretations of cases that have already come up. While the vast majority of Western democracies have constitutions that outline a priori certain conditions of government, Britain has none, preferring to muddle along on principles derived out of experience.

Thought derived of past experience is of necessity less tidy than the sweeping schemes of Cartesian thought. "English thought had always been chaos and multiplicity itself," wrote the American scholar Henry Adams early in this century.

Dr. Maurice Mercadier, a Parisian surgeon, compared the two types of thought to gardens: "The English garden is rich in a great variety of flowers chosen with taste and arranged with nonchalant elegance, whereas the French garden consists of a limited number of types of flowers, strictly selected and arranged in careful geometric patterns. The one is a harmony of colors, the other a harmony of lines. The first belongs above all to the world of the concrete, the other essentially to the world of the abstract." Margaret Mead, comparing British and American thought, wrote that the question, " 'What is your favorite color?' so intelligible to an American, is meaningless in Britain, and such a question is countered by 'Favorite color for what? A flower? A necktie?' Each object is thought of as having a most complex set of qualities, and color is merely a quality of an object, not something from a color chart on which one can make a choice which is transferable to a large number of different sorts of objects."

The Englishman likes theory in his medical thought no more than he does in his legal or political thought; nor does he like extrapolating medical findings beyond the specific cases in which they were found. For example, Professor Michael Baum explained the British position of not giving adjuvant chemotherapy in breast cancer ("adjuvant" refers to that given at the time of the original surgery or shortly afterward as an addition to the surgical treatment) in the following way: "I can understand just as well as any oncologist why it *should* work. The arguments are very persuasive. But because it ought to work doesn't mean it does. I ought to be rich, I can produce the most compelling arguments why I should be rich, yet I seem to be poor. The data are more important than the hypothesis."

According to Dr. James V. O'Brien, "From his first day as a registrar [or resident], the British registrar is liable to be plunged into the thick of the work of the specialty he aspires to join. The theory is acquired later. . . . Up to his neck from the start, he has to learn to deal with his patients as best he can—unshielded and unblinkered by theoretical considerations."

The tendency to focus on details rather than abstractions is often taken by outsiders, particularly the French, as mere pettiness. "Adam Smith studied farmers who exchanged their wheat for cloth," said Dr. Henri Pequignot, professor of internal medicine at Hôpital Cochin in Paris, "while Pierre Quesnay [a French economist] was concerned with *macroeconomics*," leaving no doubt in his tone of voice as to which approach he preferred. "English doctors are the accountants of the medical world," said another French doctor.

This respect for factual details taken together with the philosophy that the society as a whole should take precedence over the individual (a philosophy that underlies the National Health Service), explains why the British have been the chief proponents of the randomized, controlled trial in medical research, as mentioned in the "Culture Bias in Medical Science" chapter. While a Frenchman, Pierre Louis, is credited with performing the first clinical trial, trials did not become an established tradition in France—because the French did not value data collection and often had laws protecting privacy that made the collection of data impossible, there were no data to analyze. In England, on the contrary, the ideal of clinical trials meshed with the national character. The Victorian amateur scientist Francis Galton, a cousin of Darwin, created the science of biometrics, the application of probability calculus to biology. His slogan was, "Until the phenomena of any branch of knowledge have been submitted to measurement and number, it cannot assume the status and dignity of science." In his 1906 preface to *The Doctor's Dilemma,* George Bernard Shaw gave a compelling example of why clinical trials are necessary: "In Shakespear's time and for long after it, mummy was a favorite medicament. You took a pinch of the dust of a dead Egyptian in a pint of the hottest water you could bear to drink; and it did you a great deal of good. This, you thought, proved what a sovereign healer mummy was. But if you had tried the control experiment of taking the hot water without the mummy, you might have found the effect exactly the same, and that any hot drink would have done as well."

While clinical trials are becoming more widespread now in all countries, probably because they are necessary to get results published in the English-language medical literature, two differences emerge between the clinical trials conducted in England and those in America. In England, it is much more acceptable to have some of the patients receiving no treatment at all, since the English are more apt to question whether treatment of any kind is beneficial. The Medical Research Council's clinical trial of the treatment of mild hypertension, for example, included patients who received a placebo; whereas a trial of the treatment of mild hypertension in the United States compared two ways of treating the patients, since it was judged unethical not to treat patients—despite a lack of evidence that such treatment would be beneficial. Partly because the American trial did not use placebos, it is regarded as less important.

The other difference is that, once a clinical trial is complete, the British doctor will draw less sweeping conclusions from it than will the American doctor. In a recent study on the treatment of very high cholesterol with a cholesterol-lowering drug, British editorialists pointed out that results were valid only for persons treated with the same drugs for the same very high cholesterol levels used in the study. American editorialists, on the other hand, extrapolated the results of this same study from drug treatment to dietary treatment, and from patients with very high cholesterol to those with lower levels. Similarly, British doctors point out that the results of many of the trials of drugs for lowering blood pressure are only valid for men of a certain age group and only valid for the particular drugs tested. American doctors looking at the same study tend to say there is no reason to doubt that the results would be valid for everyone.

British doctors are also more likely to point out that treatment may include troubling side effects or that less medical care may actually prove to be better. For example: while American interpretations of amniocentesis trials showed the only side effects to be a slightly increased incidence of miscarriage, British trials found an increased rate of certain birth defects as well; a British trial showed that heart attack victims do as well at home as in coronary care units; and a British trial showed that pregnant women don't need more than five prenatal visits.

But if the parsimonies of British medicine are to be seen as partially resulting from a more critical medical profession, some of the economies, as well as certain excesses, must be seen more as reflections of another aspect of British character, the stiff upper lip.

British medicine, suggested Dr. Julian Leff, must be seen in light of the public-school tradition. "In the public school system, we are taught to deny the body. In the States one caters to the creature comforts." In fact, many of the criticisms of periodic examinations as well as screening tests point out that such tests will cause patients to take a morbid interest in their bodies. "In England it is doubtful if [periodic examinations] would be a success," wrote an English life insurance executive in 1928, "because we have not that large class which is found in America who have made a fortune in strenuous business and have retired while still in the prime of life, casting about for any hobby to occupy their minds. The introduction of a system of examination would concentrate people's thoughts on their internal processes and tend to perpetuate what is morbid."

Some fifty years later a letter to the *British Medical Journal* echoed the same fear: "GPs are aware that when they measure the blood pressure of a patient with a headache, on the off chance of finding a high reading, a fillip is being given to the popular association of these conditions. The interjection of a blood pressure reading willy nilly into the consultation therefore has considerable potential for spawning all manner of mischievous notions."

English patients, according to persons who have lived abroad, tend to know little about their bodies. "French people know their blood pressure," said Dr. Inch. "Not one English person in fifty knows their blood pressure." One test in 1970 showed only 42 percent of a sample of English patients could give the right location for the heart and 20 percent for the stomach.

In response to a more recent survey, Christianne Heal wrote to *Self Health*: "I work in England and Italy as a therapeutic masseuse. My Italian clients know where each organ is and understand its major functions whereas my English clients are quite as ignorant as the survey suggests."

But another writer suggested, "Although I would have got less than 40 percent on your test diagrams I am eighty-six and still going strong. Could this be because of my ignorance?"

The necessity of keeping a stiff upper lip, while accounting for the generally stoical conduct of British patients, may also explain some of the few instances where British doctors diagnose and treat more than their colleagues elsewhere. British society appears to have little tolerance for individuals who fail to maintain their self-control, and there seems to be a tendency to label such individuals sick and in need of treatment. For example, while British psychiatrists seem less likely to label patients "sick" than psychiatrists of other countries, the symptoms that they tend to overemphasize are those that indicate the patient has lost self-control. It has long been known that British psychiatrists are apt to label as manic-depressive what might be considered schizophrenia in the United States, although it seems to be the mania, rather than the depression, that really worries them.

In a comparison with U.S. psychiatrists, "UK psychiatrists tended to report more symptoms that 'overshoot the mark' such as elation, while reporting much less underactivity (dependence, indecisiveness) than did the U.S. psychiatrists." In a comparison with French and West German psychiatrists, the English were found to have much broader concepts of both neurotic and psychotic depression and of mania than did the French, with the West Germans in an intermediate position. The English psychiatrists diagnosed manic-depressive illness in 23 percent of a group of patients while the French did so in only 5 percent and the West Germans 14 percent. Analysis of the doctors' noted observations showed that the English overused the terms "agitation," "irritability," and "inability to cope with normal occupation," and underused the term "thought disorder." Among the terms overused (for the same patients) by the French were "retardation," "difficulty making decisions," "lack of energy," "passivity feelings," and "loss of normal interests."

Tranquillizer use, too, was relatively high for a country with a low overall drug use—until the NHS took action in 1984. One study, in fact, found more people taking tranquillizers over a two-week period than in any other of the countries studied. The same study showed that while 45 percent of French, German, and Spanish persons thought tranquillizers did more harm than good, and 54 percent of Italians thought the same thing, only 34 percent of English persons agreed. Another study found that while France had more prescriptions of psycholeptic and psychoanaleptic drugs in absolute terms, the UK had the greatest proportion of these drugs in its leading prescriptions.

Over 2 percent of UK prescriptions were for antidepressants. But while the English doctor appears to diagnose depression more often than his colleagues elsewhere, he apparently often treats it in such a way as to sedate the patient rather than antidepress him. Dr. Peter Tyrer, senior lecturer in psychiatry at the University of Southhampton, found that of patients referred to him by general practitioners, a quarter of the antidepressants were prescribed at doses too low to be effective as antidepressants and at that low dose would instead have a sedative effect.

Several English doctors rejected my suggestion that such a pattern of prescribing has anything to do with the British being relatively more tolerant of an oversedated patient and less tolerant of an excited one. They suggested that the overprescribing of psychoactive drugs—tranquillizers and antidepressants—for example, partly results from the fact that the GP handles persons who would be in psychotherapy in the United States; since he has little time to talk to them, he offers them drugs. In addition, since the English GP would regard vasovegetative dystonia, low blood pressure, and spasmophilia as nondiseases, he would probably label them neuroses and prescribe either uppers or downers for their sufferers rather than magnesium or spa therapy. But there is some evidence that the British patient, at least, regards taking tranquillizers as a way better to fit into British society. Cecil Helman, a GP in London who is also a social anthropologist, interviewed patients who were long-term tranquillizer users and found that over half were afraid to quit taking the drugs because of how it might affect their relationships. "In particular, they expressed fears of losing or damaging relationships due to their inability to conform to an idealized model of normal behavior and social values. A number of positive attributes were thought to be absent from the personality if the drug was not taken: these included: being normal, being oneself, even-tempered, self-controlled, patient, tolerant, good to live with, nurturing, sociable, friendly, noncomplaining, confident, popular, and being able to cope with personal and social responsibilities: 'Without it I'd be nasty, jumpy—not nice to live with.' 'I'd be unbearable to live with—all groans and moans.'

. . . Women stressed in particular the loss of their nurturing role in the family if the drug were withdrawn. Men's anxieties related to work situations and to loss of self-control.''

A similar concern about self-control may at least partially explain the British predominance in the field of anesthesiology and pain control. British anesthesiologists are highly regarded around the world and have been leaders in areas such as the development of pain clinics. There are as many anesthesiologists in Britain as there are surgeons, and no British surgeon would be allowed to operate without the services of a specialist anesthesiologist, in contrast to the situation in other countries, such as the United States, where anesthesia is sometimes given by nurse anesthetists. The English have always accepted the use of heroin both for maintenance in addicts and for pain control, and the amount used, mostly for the latter purpose, has increased markedly in the past few years. They have also created mixtures of painkilling drugs such as the Brompton cocktail—a mixture of heroin and other painkilling drugs—that have been widely adopted by other countries.

At first, the relatively high status of the fields of anesthesiology and pain relief seems a paradox in a country where the people would seem to be stoical about their bodies, and is generally attributed to the boost given to the specialty when Queen Victoria decided to have anesthesia for the birth of her eighth child. Since then, the issue of childbirth anesthesia has not been, as it has in France, whether anesthesia during childbirth should be given, but only what kind and by whom. When an analysis of causes of maternal deaths showed that some of them were due to anesthesia, the editorial writers in the *British Medical Journal* didn't suggest, as they would have in France, that anesthesia not be used, or at least not paid for by the health service, but, "There is little doubt that some anesthetic departments are not taking their obstetric duties seriously enough.''

But the high status of pain relief may not reflect that the British fear pain, but rather that they fear the loss of control that may come with pain. In the summer of 1984, for example,

I saw an English woman on television who had given birth to twins several years earlier on an Italian train. Her major concern at the time, she recalled, was that of not waking the other passengers.

For a long time, I was unable to relate another British excess—concern about their bowels—to any cultural characteristic; indeed such concern, for which there was ample evidence, seemed to contradict the general notion that the British were not supposed to pay much attention to their bodies.

"From infancy," according to an editorial in the *British Medical Journal*, "the British are brought up to regard a daily bowel action as almost a religious necessity and to believe in autointoxication from the cesspool of the unemptied colon: so it is little wonder that their doctors see vast numbers of patients obsessed with the frequency, consistency, diameter and appearance of their stools." According to another observer, Jonathan Miller in *The Body in Question*, "The English . . . are obsessed with their bowels. When an Englishman complains about constipation, you never know whether he is talking about his regularity, his lassitude, his headaches, or his depression." Probably as a consequence, a World Health Organization study found that the English had a high use of laxatives compared to other countries.

When an Englishman talks about his liver, said Dr. Dukes, he is really talking about his bowel, an observation confirmed when English patients were asked the location of various organs: 45.5 percent saw the liver as lying in the lower abdomen just above the pelvis.

Constipation perhaps really is more of a problem in England than in other countries. At least one report has shown that tea is constipating, another that the English consume more convenience foods and fewer fresh vegetables than almost any of their European Economic Community partners, and visitors to England are usually impressed by the unpalatability of the vegetables they do serve.

But the English may also perceive more constipation: 34 percent of the patients, as well as 11.4 percent of the doctors, questioned defined constipation as not opening one's bowels every day.

At least part of this obsession can be traced to the theory of autointoxication that was particularly popular in England in the early part of the twentieth century. According to the late Dr. Edward C. Lambert in *Modern Medical Mistakes*, the theory of autointoxication postulated that as a result of stasis of the intestine, the intestinal contents putrefied, forming toxins that led to chronic poisoning of the body. The attitude was exemplified in George Bernard Shaw's *The Doctor's Dilemma* by Dr. Walpole, who at one point says: " 'Ninety-five percent of the human race suffer from chronic blood-poisoning, and die of it. It's as simple as A.B.C. Your nuciform sac is full of decaying matter—undigested food and waste products—rank ptomaines. Now you take my advice, Ridgeon. Let me cut it out for you. You'll be another man afterwards. . . . I tell you this: in an intelligently governed country people wouldn't be allowed to go about with nuciform sacs, making themselves centres of infection. The operation ought to be compulsory: it's ten times more important than vaccination.' "

While the theory of autointoxication became less popular in subsequent years, it was recently revived in a slightly altered form by the English medical missionary Denis Burkitt, who has postulated that intestinal stasis leads to colon cancer. While Dr. Burkitt doesn't advocate surgery, he does advocate a high-fiber diet to produce at least daily bowel movements as the preventive. High-fiber diets, according to a comment in the *British Medical Journal*, seem "to arouse the same passions as teetotalism did in our Victorian ancestors."

The answer to my question—why this concern seems to be particularly strong in a country where the body is supposed to be denied—came in an article by Dr. Michael O'Donnell, a former editor of *World Medicine*. Dr. O'Donnell, who, having read through an "idiosyncratic A–Z of England and Englishness" found no reference to health or medicine, nurses, doctors, or patients, suggested that the medical entry for the book should be "bowels, pride in control over. Few doctors, I suspect," he wrote, "have never met the proud Englishman who, no matter how depressed he may seem during his history taking, will respond to the diffident inquiry 'bowels?' with a sunburst of triumphant smile and a defiant: 'regular as clockwork.' " Until the Second World War, wrote Dr. O'Donnell, British bowel culture was predominantly a middle-class phenomenon, but after the war "it spread rapidly through the lower orders." Dr. O'Donnell suspects that this bit of Englishness came from the public schools. Every morning at his prep school, he said, "we had to pass in line before the matron, who barked at each of us: 'Been?' and those foolish enough to answer 'No' were dosed with a foul tasting draught, which I now suspect was a mixture of rhubarb and senna."

Compared to the French and Germans, the English deemphasize *terrain*, preferring to place the cause of disease outside their body, or, failing that, in the intermediate position of their bowels. Unlike the French, British doctors do not seem to believe much in building up the resistance, and there is an almost total lack of prescription of vitamins, tonics, cures at a spa, etc. Antibiotics—drugs given against a germ—play a proportionately greater role in England. While in the West German list of the top twenty drug classes there were no antibiotics, three different classes of antibiotics made the English top twenty.

Unlike French women, who said they believed in a certain reserve of health that could be drawn upon (i.e., *terrain*), Scottish women reported they thought they were either sick or well, nothing in between. The Scottish women tended to favor as causes of disease infection, heredity and family susceptibility, and agents in the environment—specifically, poisons, working conditions, climate, or damp—and to reject natural degenerative processes or idiopathic (unknown) causes. Disease was seen as some malevolent entity residing outside the person, lying in wait to attack.

This sort of corporeal xenophobia, in fact, tends to mirror the general xenophobia of English society. Luigi Barzini has pointed out how "many Britons attributed all social disturbances to sinister outside influences. The political clashes, the high society scandals and the gruesome murders that occasionally filled the popular press were generally dismissed as 'inexplicable' mostly owing to foreign importations, to French novels or German political theories." Foreign germs have always been suspect, too, and the importation of rabies, etc., has been cited as one of the many reasons given by the English not to build a tunnel across the English Channel. Although London has fewer cases of AIDS than either Paris or New York, the British reaction to AIDS patients has been more virulent than that in France and in America, allowing local authorities to commit an AIDS patient to the hospital if they consider him a risk to others.

One favorite environmental explanation for minor illnesses in Britain is "catching a chill," used to explain all sorts of English ills from colds to bladder infections. (Perhaps British historical fear of "chills" is why most of the studies showing that air conditioning is unhealthy come from England.) Dr. Helman analyzed the responses of English patients and found that they react differently to chills than to fevers. While both attribute the cause of minor disease to something outside the body, chills signify the relationship of the body to the natural environment and fevers to social relationships, since the "bugs" that cause fevers are seen as always being carried by other people. Catching a chill in England almost always implies a certain amount of fault on the part of the patient, for example, not covering the neck with a scarf. Fevers, on the other hand, Dr. Helman found, were nobody's fault and elicited considerably more sympathy.

Chills, of course, may lead to chilblains. In contrast to some of the other "wastebasket" diagnoses I have discussed, the chilblain is unquestionably real, and consists of an itchy red blotch on the skin caused by constriction of the blood vessels due to cold—sort of an intermediate point between normalcy and frostbite. The condition exists, but is rarely diagnosed, outside of England: an international group of general practitioners left chilblains out of their classification system because they found the diagnosis was made only in England. The diagnosis, in fact, is so out of fashion in other countries that when a group of Virginia doctors found red splotches on the thighs of plump young women who rode horses in the early morning cold—classic chilblains, according to Dr. Renwick Vickers of Oxford—they thought they were describing a new disease, which they baptized "equestrian cold panniculitis."

Why are chilblains diagnosed so much more commonly in England than elsewhere?

"The English think it is immoral to heat their houses much," said Dr. Froom.

Despite the emphasis British doctors place on keeping a stiff upper lip, they are fond of saying that British medicine is kindness, not therapy, oriented. "The medical profession's blinded by the fact that they're out to cure things: cure's a mirage," said Dr. Fry. "Most common diseases are in the non-curable category. You can cure appendicitis and an infection, but you don't cure diabetes, depression, rheumatism or eczema. We are trying to relieve and comfort rather than cure."

In fact, while the British spend much less on health care than do Americans—around 6 percent of the gross national product compared to over 11 percent of our GNP, which is already much larger—their allocation of what they do have emphasizes to a much greater extent this "caring" as opposed to "therapy."

Britain is generally recognized to be ten to fifteen years ahead of Canada and the United States in geriatric medicine. The British medical system may not provide old people with high-tech treatments, but it will give them a geriatrics specialist and possibly even a psychogeriatrician. When Dr. Thomas Pickering wrote to the *British Medical Journal* pointing out that there were as many psychogeriatricians in Britain as there were cardiologists—a mistaken priority in his opinion, since he felt cardiologists could do more medically, while the job of psychogeriatrician, while important, could perhaps be better performed by social workers—a spate of responses followed, nearly all of them suggesting that life in America had corrupted *his* priorities.

Kindness can also be seen in the different interpretation often given to medical studies by the English. Not only are they more skeptical about whether medical treatment is actually doing any good; they are more sensitive to the "soft" side effects that may affect a patient's quality of life more than the hard ones. Dr. Judith Jones, a consultant in the area of international pharmaceutical laws, noted that when doctors in England and the United States were asked to report side effects of an antiulcer drug, cimetidine, the Americans tended to stick to technical side effects while the English doctors tended to pay more attention to the patient's perception of discomfort, noting the more subjective side effects such as confusion. A British reviewer of a book on cancer chemotherapy noted that in the six hundred-page book there "is too much uncritical listing of drugs found to be 'active' (this so-called activity sometimes achieving very little of real benefit to the patient) and too little discussion of what side effects may mean to the patient and his family, especially psychological effects. The quality of life is hardly mentioned."

The lesser belief in medicine's ability to prolong life and the greater belief in medicine's role in making life nicer are undoubtedly the reason that hospices for the dying grew up first in Britain, not America. To accept the idea of hospice, one must accept the fact that people die, and "in the UK we strive less officiously to keep alive. This is not callousness but stems from a different attitude to death. American physicians seem to regard death as the ultimate failure of their skill. British doctors frequently regard death as physiological, sometimes even devoutly to be wished," Dr. Hull wrote.

"There is a fit between hospice and the British temper that does not seem to exist in America," wrote two observers of the British hospice system in the *Hastings Center Report*. "The British ethos has suffered through two wars in ways Americans can't imagine, and it is an ethos in which acceptance of finitude or mortality—the crucial precondition for hospice's success—is more widespread. It's not by accident that the British started hospices long before we did."

But the caring is often paternalistic, and the British patient probably has fewer rights than his counterpart in France, West Germany, or the United States. Patients can be involuntarily committed to a hospital more easily, either because they have an infectious disease like AIDS or because of a psychiatric defect; and the right of a patient to be informed of the risks of medical procedures was recently denied by the British House of Lords, shocking medical-legal experts in West Germany and France. Moreover, the comforting is often more what the doctor thinks the patient wants than what the patient may actually want. When Jean Robinson entered the hospital for an operation and was given a consent form to sign, she said, "I told the sister I couldn't sign it because it said I had been told the nature and purpose of the procedure and I hadn't been. They then called in the anesthetist, who said they would give me an extra shot. Requests for information are regarded as a need for reassurance."

One study found that 33 percent of British patients did not question the doctor because they thought he would think less of them, and 20 percent were scared they would get a bad or hostile reaction. However, 80 percent of the patients who did ask clear-cut questions received specific answers. Patients are allowed to change GPs only with difficulty, and a request to change doctors is viewed more as a sign of patient deviance than anything else. While in theory one can change doctors at any time, "in practice it doesn't work like that. Any doctor is very suspicious of patients who change doctors and in some areas they have a gentleman's agreement not to take each other's patients," said Ms. Robinson. Asked what he would do if a patient didn't like a specialist to whom he had been referred, Dr. Fry said, "I would change the specialist, but I might warn him that the patient hadn't gotten on with his predecessor."

Such curbs on personal liberty would be taken very badly in the United States. But we can certainly learn from the more critical questioning of British doctors as to whether they are actually doing their patients any good. The English medical literature can provide us with a valuable source of second opinions, being somewhat franker about "soft" side effects as well as showing us that treatments regarded by American doctors as effective are often regarded in England as only marginally so. As a corollary, if British doctors believe something works, we can be reasonably confident that it does.

United States:
The Virus in the Machine

> In short, as I have said, he was healthy, normal and happy. And
> then, one fatal day at his club, he heard of the Health Audit.
> The idea (I fall into the lingo of Service) Appealed to him
> Instantly.
> He was going to have his Health Audited.
> Would he let his business go a year without having an Audit? He
> would Not!
> Would he let his automobile run three months without an
> Overhauling? No.
> Was his Body less important than his automobile? . . .
> Now he insists in conversation that the health audit lengthened
> his life ten years, though he has lived only two and a half since it
> was made, and he intends to be audited again next year.
> —Dr. Logan Clendening,
> *The Care and Feeding of Adults*

Even as Europeans were developing the simple mastectomy
and the lumpectomy as less mutilating ways to treat breast
cancer, American doctors were advocating the superradical
mastectomy and prophylactic removal of both breasts to prevent
breast cancer.

American medicine is aggressive. From birth—which is more
likely to be by cesarean than anywhere in Europe—to death in
hospital, from invasive examination to prophylactic surgery,
American doctors want to *do* something, preferably as much as
possible. As the medical house officer created by Dr. Samuel

124

Shem in his book *The House of God* said, "I'm the captain of this ship, and I deliver medical care, which, for your information, means not doing nothing, but doing something. In fact, doing everything you can, see?"

American doctors perform more diagnostic tests than doctors in France, West Germany, or England. They often eschew drug treatment in favor of more aggressive surgery, but if they do use drugs they are likely to use higher doses and more aggressive drugs. While official recommendations as to dose are often higher than those given in other countries, even when official recommendations drop many doctors continue to believe that higher doses will be better. When, for example, the recommended dosage of anticoagulants was lowered, many doctors continued to use the higher dosages, even though such doses increased the danger of bleeding.

The dosages in psychiatry are particularly high, sometimes as much as ten times those used elsewhere. "I think we use higher drug doses than anybody in the world except maybe the Russians," said Dr. Jonathan O. Cole of McLean Hospital in Belmont, Massachusetts. "We try to declare chemical warfare on psychosis."

Surgery, too, besides being performed more often, is likely to be more aggressive when it is performed. This seems to be particularly true where surgery on or near the sex organs is performed. An American woman has two to three times the chance of having a hysterectomy as her counterpart in England, France, or West Germany, and foreign doctors joke about American "birthday hysterectomies" perhaps without realizing how young the birthday is: over 60 percent of hysterectomies in the United States are performed in women under forty-four. Besides the policy of some doctors of taking out uteruses routinely in healthy women around the age of forty, often with removal of the ovaries, too, a policy approved by the 1975 edition of one of the leading gynecologic textbooks, many U.S. doctors consider hysterectomy the treatment for many precancerous conditions treated less radically in Europe. When cancer is found, the surgery will be more radical. Prostate surgery also will be performed more often than in Europe, and will be performed on both younger and older men. America is perhaps the only country outside of Israel where a majority of male infants are still routinely circumcised.

Public health policies on vaccination will often be aimed at eliminating the disease, not, as is true elsewhere, at protecting individuals. When the vaccine for rubella came on the market, for example, most European countries vaccinated only prepubertal girls; the United States vaccinated all children in an attempt to wipe out the disease—quickly.

Many conditions, such as high blood pressure, are diagnosed and treated aggressively. Even before the Hypertension Detection and Follow-up Program was published in the *Journal of the American Medical Association* in 1979, giving some justification for the treatment of mildly raised blood pressure, some American doctors were using "an approach more aggressive than could be justified by the then available evidence concerning the relative benefits and hazards of treating mild hypertensives."

Even when American medicine leans toward the "gentle" therapies it does so using aggressive language, and the word "aggressive" is used so often regarding the screening, diagnosis, and treatment of diseases that one suspects it confers a particular psychological satisfaction. When American blood pressure experts announced in 1984 what was essentially a policy of retrenchment, reversing an earlier recommendation for aggressive drug treatment of even mild hypertension, they urged that nondrug therapies such as diet, exercise, and behavior modification be "pursued aggressively."

And when a twelve-hospital study of the treatment of premature infants found that those at one hospital had been treated more gently and had fewer complications (interestingly, their treatment was supervised by a Chinese doctor) than those at the eleven other hospitals, the author of the study did not recommend that the gentler treatments be adopted nationwide but instead called for further research. Further research is always commendable, but one wonders whether it would be called for had the results shown more aggressive treatment was associated with a better outcome.

This medical aggressiveness reflects an aggressiveness of the American character that has often been attributed to the effect the vast frontier had on the people (mostly Europeans) who came to settle it. The once seemingly limitless lands gave rise to a spirit that anything was possible if only the natural environment, with its extremes of weather, poisonous flora and fauna, and the sometimes unfriendly native Americans, could be conquered. Disease also could be conquered, but only by aggressively ferreting it out diagnostically and just as aggressively treating it, preferably by taking something out rather than adding something to increase the resistance. Disease might even be prevented by cleansing the environment of hostile elements. As Oliver Wendell Holmes put it: "How could a people which has a revolution once in four years, which has contrived the Bowie knife and the revolver . . . which insists in sending out yachts and horses and boys to outsail, outrun, outfight and checkmate all the rest of creation; how could such a people be content with any but 'heroic' practice? What wonder that the stars and stripes wave over doses of ninety grains of sulphate of quinine and that the American eagle screams with delight to see three drachms [180 grains] of calomel given at a single mouthful?"

The aggressive approach that has characterized American medicine was evident even before the American revolution. Dr. Benjamin Rush, one of the signers of the Declaration of Independence and a doctor whose influence on American medicine lasted for decades, believed that one of the hindrances to the development of medicine had been an "undue reliance upon the powers of nature in curing disease," a thesis he blamed on Hippocrates. John Duffy, a professor of history at the University of Maryland and author of *The Healers*, explained that Rush was converted to aggressive medicine during a yellow-fever epidemic, when he found that larger and larger quantities of mercury and jalap (purges) appeared to cure the patients. While Duffy suggests that these particular patients had not had yellow fever, or only mild cases, "Whatever the case, Rush became convinced that he had solved the problem. . . . Rush's success in promulgating his thesis meant that for many years to come massive purging and bloodletting were to characterize American medical practice." Rush "believed that the body held about 25 pints of blood, over double the actual quantity, and he urged his disciples to continue bleeding until four-fifths of the body's blood was removed. When massive purging caused the bowels to bleed, he felt the purge was doing double duty." Rush was imbued with the idea that even nature itself had been put under control of the American Revolution.

Another historian, Martin S. Pernick, says that "Rush promoted his therapies in part by convincing practitioners and patients alike that they were heroic, bold, courageous, manly, and patriotic. Americans were tougher than Europeans; American diseases were correspondingly tougher than mild European diseases; to cure Americans would require uniquely powerful doses administered by heroic American physicians."

By the early nineteenth century Rush's approach was epitomized by a phrase one finds repeatedly in medical journals of the day: "desperate diseases require desperate remedies." In Louisiana, according to Duffy, while the Creole physicians believed the role of the physician was to assist nature in making the cure, "the Anglo-American doctors generally espoused the doctrines of Benjamin Rush, scorning the healing power of nature and firmly believing in direct and drastic interferences. When confronted by a sick patient, they gathered their purges and emetics, couched their lancets, and charged the enemy, prepared to bleed, purge and vomit until the disease was conquered."

Pernick cites a popular medical author from Cincinnati who wrote that "mildness of medical treatment is real cruelty." What was needed, the author declared, was a "vigorous mode of practice; the diseases of our own country especially require it."

Pernick notes that " 'Frontier' surgeons like Ephraim Mc-
Dowell, Nathan Smith, and J. Marion Sims developed new operations which, they bragged, Europeans had been too sensitive
and timid to perform. . . . American surgeons attributed their
successes in part to a frontier stoicism lacking in effete Old World
practitioners; European critics denounced the American practice
as an example of frontier barbarism and cruelty."

When France became the mecca of medical progress in the
mid-nineteenth century, a number of American physicians, including Oliver Wendell Holmes, studied there and some of them,
like Holmes, brought home the cause of moderation. But most
were more selective about what they brought. While they admired the diagnostic prowess of the French, they distrusted the
"therapeutic nihilism" there. Historian John Harley Warner found
that most Americans studying in France at that time thought
French medicine was characterized by a distrust of the efficacy
of remedies and an expectant method of treatment that gave
primacy to the healing power of nature. The imperative to in-
tervene was critical to American physicians' professional iden-
tity, and to them the therapeutic skepticism of French doctors
seemed to imply a "do-nothing" plan of practice and an ab-
negation of professional responsibility. Warner wrote: "Although a non-interventionist plan might perhaps be suited to
the inmates of Parisian hospitals (and of this Americans had
their doubts), most Amerian physicians agreed that it was not
appropriate for American circumstances, which demanded active treatment."

The tendency to favor aggressive therapy, and to mistrust
nature, has remained into the twentieth century. The almost
universal use of episiotomy in childbirth, for example, can be
traced to Dr. Joseph DeLee, an obstetrician who in 1920 recommended the routine use of forceps, episiotomy, and the early
removal of the placenta. An artificial cut, argued DeLee, was so
much cleaner and more controlled than a jagged, natural tear.
Nurse and writer Margarete Sandelowski points out that DeLee
revealed his abhorrence of natural labor best when he stated

that he often wondered " 'whether Nature did not deliberately intend women to be used up in the process of reproduction, in a manner analogous to that of the Salmon which dies after spawning.' "

Sandelowski also says that "DeLee mused that it was probably better for the health of the infant if all deliveries were by cesarean section rather than allowing it to struggle through the torturous passages of its mother's beleaguered genital tract."

DeLee eventually had second thoughts about the role he had played in promoting the cause of prophylactic obstetrics when such practices were shown to be a major cause of birth-related accidents. But aggressive obstetrics accorded too much with American values to be routed by mere second thoughts: by the 1980s episiotomy continued to be almost universal in American deliveries, with the cesarean section rate climbing to above 20 percent even though the neonatal death rate remained higher than that of Europe, with its much lower cesarean section rates. Even with widespread calls to limit the rate of cesarean sections, the rates continued to climb in the mid-1980s.

Cesarean section is now the most commonly performed operation in the United States; hysterectomy is the second most common, and the same abhorrence of nature undoubtedly lies behind the preference for hysterectomy. Dr. Ralph C. Wright, for example, has argued that "After the last planned pregnancy, the uterus becomes a useless, bleeding, symptom-producing, potentially cancer-bearing organ and therefore should be removed." Wright added: "If, in addition, both ovaries are removed, further benefits accrue," failing to mention that removal of both ovaries without artificially replacing the ovarian hormones causes a variety of diseases and results in a higher death rate than had they not been removed. While Wright is often cited as an extreme case, the widely used *Novak's Textbook of Gynecology* in its 1975 edition noted that "Menstruation is a nuisance to most women, and if this can be abolished without impairing ovarian function, it would probably be a blessing to not only the woman but to her husband. . . . Thus one can make a rather convincing case for the value of elective hysterectomy, and there seems definitely a trend in this community, as well as in the country as a whole for this to be the procedure of choice."

An aggressive approach, of course, implies that the doctor can do something for the patients, and this "can-do" attitude is as much a characteristic of American medicine as it is of the American character in general.

"Pragmatic Americans," wrote Luigi Barzini in *The Europeans*, "consider the very existence of problems intolerable and life with problems unacceptable. They believe . . . that all problems not only must be solved, but also that they can be solved, and that in fact the main purpose of a man's life is the solution of problems." This means that Americans tend to feel it is better to do something rather than not do anything. "I call them the 'Godsakers,' " said the English Dr. Fry. " 'For God's sake *do* something.' "

All this trying to do something results in a rushing about both of Americans in general and of their doctors. Barzini observed that "for more than two centuries foreign visitors to the United States noticed with awe that the inhabitants were all anxiously rushing about, always in a great hurry, and many of them, like Thomas Jefferson, were tirelessly inventing time-saving devices." One author has called American medicine "Obsessive-Compulsive," and the British medical student Dr. Eleanor Moskovic, who spent some time at Massachusetts General Hospital, noted, "There seemed to be an overwhelming number of so-called 'type A' personalities around—and the only explanation I could offer for this was that American medicine selects, and is selected by a different type of student than in England. 'Big' money and a position of enormous social and academic prestige are conferred on successful American doctors—perhaps it therefore attracts 'business men' who react to it as they would to private enterprise." Still another British observer come to do a residency in America wrote that "sometimes at 6:30 in the morning the bones ache a little and I think wistfully of gentle 8:30 ward rounds followed by tea and biscuits in sister's office."

The can-do attitude has, of course, its advantages. America has essentially eliminated measles within its borders—something many other developed countries have not achieved—although cases are still contracted from persons abroad. The emphasis on medical research has resulted in a number of Nobel Prize–winning discoveries that benefit people all over the world. Technological innovations such as CAT scanners are made widely available, and while they are undoubtedly overused, in many cases they provide diagnosis more comfortably and effectively than did older methods. Perhaps most dramatically, the American rate of heart attack has fallen by 40 percent in the past twenty years, and while doctors dispute whether this has been due to treatment or prevention, both were undertaken aggressively.

But all this rushing about aggressively to do something can also take its toll upon the American health. Neurasthenia, or nervous exhaustion, was at first called "the American Disease." The French psychiatrist Charcot in 1887 described neurasthenic Americans who today might be said to be suffering from "burnout": "It is actually true that many Americans have a way of working which is peculiarly their own: once they have set themselves a task, they stick to it stubbornly for a considerable period of time which sometimes runs into years. They go to extremes, they make it a matter of pride, nothing distracts them, and after a certain time, they fall a prey to neurasthenia. After so much work their poor brain refuses to function any longer."

Another victim of the can-do approach in American medicine is the patient who can't, or won't, do anything about his or her condition. One psychiatric observer, for example, found that the calm and placid patients and their families were more likely to be considered sick, and that frequent activity, even meaningless activity, was preferred to thought, and desperate cheerfulness to calm acceptance.

Similarly, the patient who "beats" cancer is considered su-

perior to the patient who fights but succumbs, who is in turn
superior to the patient who refuses to fight.

"When you refer to one group of people as 'victors,' what
would you call the others," wrote the daughter of a cancer
victim to *The New York Times Magazine* in response to an article
about people who had "beaten cancer." The implication of the
article, she said, was "that 'winning' against cancer is some sort
of holy crusade, and that victory is simply a matter of will. What,
then, is he implying about those who fought back but did not
'conquer'?" Dr. Perri Klass points out that if a patient gets worse
following chemotherapy, that patient is said to have "failed"
chemotherapy.

Those who refuse treatment entirely, even when their case
is hopeless, are considered deviant, and are often hauled into
court. When William Bartling, suffering from five potentially
fatal diseases including an inoperable lung cancer, at the age of
seventy wanted to have his ventilator taken away, the judge
characterized Mr. Bartling's prognosis for recovery as "guarded
and cautious, but optimistic" and ordered that he remain on
the respirator and would not order that his hands be untied.

That a man with five potentially fatal diseases can be considered as having an "optimistic" prognosis if only he is forced
to take a treatment reveals perhaps the most troubling aspect
of the American can-do approach, that the risks of treatment
are often underestimated while the risks of no treatment are
often overestimated.

Dr. Klass, writing of her Harvard Medical School education,
says, "As a medical student, I knew I was being trained to rely
heavily on technology, to assume that the risk of acting is almost
always preferable to the risk of not acting. . . . My class in medical school was absorbing the idea that when it comes to tests,
technology and interventions, more is better. No one ever talked
about the negative aspects of intervention, and the one time a
student asked about the 'appropriateness' of fetal monitoring,
the question was cut off with a remark that there was no time
to discuss issues of 'appropriateness.' "

The same clinical trials that will be interpreted cautiously in England are often touted in the United States as definitive proof that treatment works. One trial of the treatment of mild hypertension, for example, was interpreted as showing that proper treatment reduced mortality by 20 percent, but an English-born blood pressure expert, Dr. Thomas Pickering of New York Hospital, pointed out that in fact the mortality in the treated group was 6.4 percent and in the control group 7.7 percent, an actual difference of 1.3 percent. "Thus, for every 100 patients treated, 1.3 derived benefit and 98.7 did not." In fact this trial was widely criticized by the English on the grounds that there was no group that did not receive some treatment: American doctors were so certain mild hypertension should be treated they did not feel it was ethical not to treat some patients, even though it had not yet been shown whether such treatment did them more good than harm.

When pressed as to whether aggressive treatment is really better, American doctors often answer that they must treat aggressively or they will get sued for malpractice. There is some evidence in support of this: American (as well as English) law tends to require that everything possible be done for the patient, and doctors certainly believe that juries will be kinder on their sins of commission than on their sins of omission.

The threat of malpractice combined with the penchant of national bodies such as the American Heart Association to recommend aggressive treatments often influences doctors' recommendations. When an internist I was seeing for the first time finally diagnosed as a mitral valve prolapse the heart murmur other internists had been hearing for years, he told me I should take antibiotics whenever I had any dental procedure whatsoever, including having my teeth cleaned. To me, this recommendation seemed to combine two quintessential American culture values: the corporeal xenophobia we share with the English that the disease (in this case the bacteria liberated into the bloodstream during dental procedures) is more important than the *terrain*, which in this case was the ability of my immune system to handle the bacteria on its own, and the American belief that it is better to do something than not to do something. I therefore suspected that antibiotics were being recommended without much evidence of benefit. A trip to the medical library convinced me I was right—the literature made clear that researchers did not know whether the risks of taking antibiotics exceeded the extremely low risk for patients like myself of developing endocarditis. The recommendation was being made on the grounds that, in the face of unknown risks and benefits, it was better to do something than to do nothing.

I wrote a letter to my dentist explaining that while I was aware of the slight risk involved, I refused to take antibiotics for minor dental procedures because I believed in such a situation it is better not to do anything at all. I sent a copy to the internist, who later told me he agreed with me, but felt he had to prescribe antibiotics since the American Heart Association had so recommended.

To make certain I was really dealing with American culture bias, I later passed this incident by a French professor of medicine to see what the practice in France would be. He explained that for the third and most severe grade of mitral valve prolapse a French doctor *might* prescribe antibiotics for a patient having a tooth pulled. But what about for a patient having his teeth cleaned, which was the recommendation in the United States? The French doctor seemed puzzled. Why would anyone with healthy teeth go to the dentist once or twice a year to have their teeth cleaned? he wondered.

While doctors may feel that aggressive treatment will be a better defense in a malpractice case, it is less certain that aggressive treatment is better for the patient, since treatment may lead to side effects more serious than the original disease.

In one university hospital, 36 percent of patients had an iatrogenic (treatment-caused) disease, that in one-fourth of them was either life-threatening or produced considerable disability and in 2 percent was believed to contribute to the death of the patient. This figure probably errs on the conservative side, noted the authors. They did not count: complications if there was any chance that they were due to the disease, not to the treatment; obviously minor events; or side effects that could not be documented, even though the staff felt they were due to treatment. Cancer patients, who are particularly prone to treatment side effects, were not included in the study. Whether such events are more common in the United States than elsewhere cannot yet be proven, but most observers believe more aggressive treatment is associated with a higher rate of side effects.

"In France," said hepatologist Jean-Pierre Benhamou, "we use ineffective medicines in an ineffective manner. In the States, you use effective medicines in an ineffective manner." As a result, he said, therapeutic accidents are more frequent in the United States, because the drugs are stronger.

A group led by Nathan Couch at Peter Bent Brigham Hospital in Boston analyzed surgical errors over a one-year period, and found that, in two-thirds of the cases, adverse outcomes were due to errors of commission, not of omission. When they analyzed why the errors had occurred, they found a group of typically American thought processes. Some of the errors were due to misplaced optimism: for example, an overestimation of surgical skill with an underestimation of the patient's fragility. Other errors were due to unwarranted urgency: for example, extensive surgery in seriously ill cancer patients that could not possibly cure the patient and in fact shortened an already limited life. Still others arose from the urge for perfection, which resulted in wide-ranging operative manipulation considerably beyond the level needed for relief of the patient's most important problem; and still others from the performance of new stylish procedures, including the recent trend toward a return to superradical cancer resection.

And while the can-do approach has been cited in cutting the U.S. rate of heart attack and stroke, as well as virtually eliminating certain infectious diseases, some diseases have not proven so amenable to the aggressive approach. In spite of declarations of war on cancer and predictions dating back at least fifty years that a cure is just around the corner, death rates from cancer have actually been rising. This lack of progress has not, however, caused Americans to doubt that cancer *can* be cured. As Senator George McGovern put it, "I have a suspicion that we're losing the war on cancer because of mistaken priorities and misallocation of funds."

Defeats never seem to call into doubt that aggressive approach; in fact, they simply give rise to more aggressive approaches. In the face of rising death rates from breast cancer, Americans call for more aggressive screening, in spite of the fact that there is not much evidence that screening of women under the age of fifty will prolong their survival. The failure of a low-fat diet to prevent breast cancer metastases in a short-term follow-up simply caused doctors to say that the diets were not low enough in fat.

Americans not only want to *do* something, they want to do it *fast*, and if they cannot they often become frustrated. "Americans are not very good at handling chronic situations," said Dr. Zarday, the internist born in Hungary, educated in Germany, and now practicing in New York City. "They want immediate results, in medicine as well as in everything else. I always get amused at a certain type of American newspaper headline— 'Relief Sent to Africa But Starvation Continues'—that assumes that situations like starvation can be handled overnight."

As a consequence, in the opinion of many, Americans are not very good at treating chronic diseases. "Chronic diseases such as chronic bronchitis and chronic rheumatism are not well treated in the United States," said Professor Jan J. de Blecourt, a rheumatologist in Groningen, the Netherlands. "Only diseases causing death and infections are considered important in the United States." A reflection of this bias can be seen in the way medical insurance reimburses doctors and patients for illness. In contrast to the situation in Europe, where all illness, whether acute or chronic, is taken care of, in the United States, Medicare will assume responsibility only for diseases considered "curable," leaving patients with chronic, incurable conditions such as Alzheimer's disease out in the cold. Rehabilitation, too, is a poor stepchild of American medicine, and in the case of stroke, patients must possess two typically American qualities: "recovery potential" and "motivation" even to be accepted into many rehabilitation programs.

One problem, of course, is that there are no medical spas in the United States; and spas, all questions about the curative values of their waters aside, have evolved in continental Europe into treatment centers for chronic diseases. One state department official whose wife contracted multiple sclerosis while he was stationed in East Germany said that her treatment seemed to be better in Czechoslovakia and East Germany than in the United States. Her physical therapy was more rigorous at the Czech spa of Piestanny and she began to walk again there. By contrast, when she got back to the States and was put into Georgetown Hospital in Washington she developed a number of problems, including bedsores.

"My wife definitely felt that the more vigorous physical therapy received in Czechoslovakia was more useful," said the official, who preferred to be unnamed. "Here the therapist is always on a time schedule." Doctors in the United States, he found, favored the use of physical therapy but really didn't think it did much for the disease. In East Germany, by contrast, he said, the therapist would come at two and stay until five—would sit and chat and have a cup of coffee and bring her children. "The benefit might have been psychological," the official admitted, for his wife felt more interest was being taken in her case.

The penchant for doing things fast also means that surgical procedures that may have to be repeated are not looked upon kindly. Regarding fibroid tumors of the uterus, American doctors I interviewed emphasized that myomectomy, the operation that removed the fibroids but left in the uterus, might have to be repeated; several of the doctors exaggerated the risk of recurrence, with the implication that myomectomy was therefore a procedure to be avoided in favor of hysterectomy. (Myomectomy also often takes longer than hysterectomy.) None of the French doctors I talked to even mentioned recurrence, probably because they felt it was a small price to pay for keeping one's uterus. When I asked, I was told they felt in France that six myomectomies could be performed before the patient would even require a cesarean section if she became pregnant! Similar arguments about recurrence are used against the synovectomy, a treatment for arthritis.

Similarly, studies of what works and what doesn't are often evaluated in the short term. Drugs, for example, may appear to be more effective for schizophrenia than psychotherapy, but this may be simply because they work faster. When President Reagan had his prostate operation, the mortality statistics for the operation cited were very low, since they had taken into account only those deaths that occurred during and immediately after the operation. A study that followed patients for up to a year found that, in fact, the operated patients had a higher death rate for several months following the operation.

The American regards himself as naturally healthy. It therefore stands to reason that if he becomes ill, there must be a cause for the illness, preferably one that comes from without and can be quickly dealt with.

Probably as a result, Americans have developed a passion for diagnosis. As Dr. Samuel Shem wrote of medical students, "They all shared the belief that disease was some wild and hairy monster to be locked up in the neat medical grids of differential diagnosis and treatment. All it took was a little superhuman effort and all would be well."

Alistair Cooke notes that in even the most distinguished British biographies of literary figures, musicians, and artists, five hundred pages of the most scrupulous scholarship will end with the note that "the great man or woman tired easily, was in increasing pain, and friends knew that 'the end was near.' " Nearly fifty years previously, Cooke noted, his first American friend, then a premedical student at Yale, on coming to the end of a biography of some writer said: " 'What *is* this listlessness that killed him? Was it an anaemia, diabetes, encephalitis, or what?' . . . The American internist expects to be burdened by this nagging demand—from a lawyer, a housewife, an actor, or a real estate broker—for a technical explanation that would bore or bewilder the more stoical Briton." Young journalists in America are taught never to write in an obituary that someone died of "natural" causes, apparently because death is never considered natural but rather due to something external. They are taught it is better to find out the cause of death—even though numerous studies have shown that the cause of death on the death certificate often doesn't correlate with the cause of death if an autopsy is performed.

The search for a diagnosis means, in America, tests, since American doctors are not particularly known for their clinical skills in examining the patient. This tendency was already apparent to foreign visitors in the early 1900s. As Stanley Joel Reiser relates in *Medicine and the Reign of Technology*, when the British physician Sir Humphrey Rolleston visited the United States on a tour of medical facilities in 1908, he pointed out what he considered the American physician's serious inattention to bedside observation and examination of the patient. Four years later, a Parisian physician touring American hospitals reported his surprise at the number of laboratory tests routinely requested for the patients. To him, the tests seemed "like the Lord's rain, to descend from Heaven on the just and on the unjust in the most impartial fashion," and he concluded that "the diagnosis and treatment of a given patient depended more on the result of these various tests than on the symptoms present in the case."

A patient seeing a GP in the United States will have more tests than would the patient seeing the GP in practically any European country. In addition, a U.S. patient is likely to see an internist, who gives even more tests.

In hospital, too, the patient will have more tests, including more invasive ones. In a study of hospitals in several European countries, Dr. Steven A. Schroeder found that "all other things being equal, a patient in the U.S. university hospital will have more diagnostic tests and therapies performed. This seems to hold true to 'little ticket' items such as blood chemistry tests and intravenous therapy as well as for 'big ticket' categories such as ultrasound or coronary bypass surgery, or telemetry monitoring." Another comparison, this one between intensive care units in France and the United States, showed similar results.

Eleanor Moskovic, the British doctor who spent some time at Massachusetts General Hospital when she was a medical student, found that "the patients on the whole saw many more 'procedures' than their English counterparts. Many of the myocardial infarcts were 'cath-ed' routinely, few patients escaped a daily X-ray examination, most had ultrasound of something at some stage, daily Pan-scans, of course, and lots of blood gases—for which there seemed to be a particularly low threshold. Computed tomography scanning was extremely popular— I was told by one resident that it was very accurate in the diagnosis of sinusitis."

Many Americans, of course, believe that more tests of necessity indicate better medicine. But many observers of American medicine don't agree. Dr. Donald Young, of the Mayo Clinic's department of biochemistry, speaking at the forty-eighth annual meeting of the Royal College of Physicians and Surgeons in Canada, said most tests were "fishing trips looking for something wrong when there's no justification." He suggested that 75 percent of diagnoses can be made by the physician directly interviewing the patient, a physical exam probably yields another 15 to 20 percent results, and laboratory tests, ECGs, etc., account for only 5 to 10 percent input into the eventual diagnosis.

"I am convinced," wrote Dr. Mike Oppenheim in the *New England Journal of Medicine*, "that Americans experience a mystical, atavistic satisfaction in handing over a small amount of their blood to a physician and hearing a few days later the solemn announcement: 'everything was normal.' In fact, no blood test or X-ray study performed regularly in a person who feels well is useful in detecting hidden, treatable disease."

Not only is such testing expensive, taking resources away from other areas, such as treatment of chronic diseases; it can also cause side effects. And such aggressive diagnosing often sets the stage for aggressive therapy. Electronic fetal monitoring, for example, has been shown to increase the rate of cesarean sections threefold, with no measurable benefit to either mother or baby. One obstetrician explained that electronic fetal monitoring is performed while the patient is in bed, and being in bed can lead to uterine dysfunction. Oxytocin is given to correct uterine dysfunction and the monitor registers signs interpreted as fetal distress, which leads to a decision for a cesarean.

Similarly, the frequent screening by Pap smears for cervical cancer may lead to more aggressive therapy. Recommendations for the interval between screens is now one to three years, still much closer than the British once every five years. Many U.S. doctors, however, continue to recommend Pap smears every six months, and if the smear is slightly abnormal, it will probably be treated more aggressively in America than elsewhere, sometimes by hysterectomy.

A California physician explained: "The recommendation that all women get their Pap test is even on television now. So patients come in for a test because everybody else does it. You may not be concerned with that in England, but in the United States we're stuck with doing Pap smears on many young women and once we get an abnormal report we've got to take care of it."

When all this aggressive diagnosis and treatment became too expensive for a system in which doctors are paid for each act they perform, reforms were started, and the reforms, too, had a distinctly American air. Rather than reimbursing physicians for everything they did, reimbursement would be based on the diagnosis the patient was given. Such a system gives primacy to the idea that disease is some wild and hairy monster that can be locked up with diagnosis, and completely ignores the European idea that the severity of disease—and consequently the need for medical intervention—has also to do with features such as *terrain*.

If, in spite of all the tests, doctors are not able to come up with any abnormalities, in the United States the favored "wastebasket explanation" is a virus, alias low-grade virus. "What doctors don't know, they attribute to a virus, or when a condition doesn't respond to treatment, they attribute it to a virus," said Dr. Iwao Moriyama, a longtime director of the U.S. National Center for Health Statistics.

Alistair Cooke, in an article in the *British Medical Journal*, noted of the "magic word" *virus*: "All suffering people drop it to explain a sniffle or a sleepiness. . . . I used it myself freely till, to my shame, a doctor present said something like: 'I don't think it's a virus. I doubt it has protein coat.' " "America has an overall virus mentality," said the West German Dr. Viefhues. According to Robert Abrahams, a professor of folklore at the University of Pennsylvania, people protect themselves as a group and as individuals from malevolent forces. "In some societies it is witches. For Americans, it is germs."

"Infectious diseases," according to Dr. Zarday, "appeal to Americans because they can be conquered easily and immediately. An infection is purely external—no part of you. That's one reason Americans have had enormous success in infectious diseases."

In America, the presence of a virus (or of bacteria) is emphasized with little play given to host resistance. Doctors often cite the study of islanders who didn't develop a particular disease until foreigners came to the island, which they claim, truthfully, is proof that one cannot get a viral disease in the absence of a virus. French and West German doctors would point out that while a virus may be necessary for the development of a viral disease, resistance obviously plays a role, since not everyone exposed gets the disease.

So strong is the belief that germs, and only germs, are important in the cause of disease that when a woman wrote to *Fortune* magazine saying that no one in her family had had a cold or the flu in a dozen years because they ate fresh garlic and onions regularly, four persons answered, all suggesting that the garlic and onions were doing their job only by preventing human contact. One wrote: "Those are communicable diseases passed by contact from one person to another. I'd guess that during that dozen years no one in her family had a baby, either."

While West German doctors would maintain that an antibiotic should be given only if the infection was caused by a bacteria *and* was also serious, American doctors are content to prescribe an antibiotic simply if a bacteria is present. In fact, many are content if a bacteria is possibly present, and this probably explains in part why antibiotic use in the United States is so high: one comparison found American doctors prescribed about twice as many antibiotics as Scottish doctors; and, as we have already seen, the United Kingdom has a higher use of antibiotics than does West Germany.

American medical researchers, too, often seem to believe that all will be solved once a virus is found in association with a disease; and such an association is always cause for great to-do in the press. The federal War Against Cancer program initially put most of its funding into finding a viral cause of cancer. Recently, Dr. Zarday said he had been quite surprised at publicity about a child who had developed diabetes following a viral infection. "The problem is not that it's one case, but that it's only an association, and associations should be statistical. I don't think if we find a virus all our problems are solved."

The idea that disease must be caused by something in the environment, probably a germ, can explain the American penchant for cleanliness. Most foreigners find amusing the lengths Americans go to keep themselves and everything around them clean. Of all the foreigners visiting France, claimed one French woman, "it is the Americans who will not drink the water, and if they do, they are the only ones who will get sick." After

World War II, said the West German Dr. Naumann, "we admired the amount of cleaning activity of the American military families. They were always boiling water and they used large amounts of cleaning chemicals—everything had to be disinfected. We found this kind of astonishing."

In an advertisement for one antiseptic cleanser, Americans are told, "If you could see the germs, you would use it every day." Americans are warned to avoid kissing and other contact with family members who may have a cold, with one article going so far as to say such avoidance would help build up resistance, when in fact the opposite is true. An article that concluded scientifically that even dirty toilet seats were probably not a hazard for a healthy person nevertheless mentioned several tips that included avoiding touching the toilet seat, tossing the first circle of toilet paper, flushing with a foot instead of a bare hand, and turning off the faucet, after hand washing, with a paper towel.

The medical profession itself is probably less convinced than the public at large that such fastidiousness is necessary for health: "We look too much at aesthetics," said Dr. Kruse. "We're doing what people want. We spend a lot of effort looking for cockroaches or hairs, which have a very limited effect on health."

Said Dr. Mafouz Zaki, a public health official for Long Island, New York: "We recommend that hair [of restaurant workers] is kept clean and covered mostly for aesthetic reasons. If you're paying fifteen dollars for a meal, you don't like to get blond hair coming out of your soup."

The American penchant for cleanliness undoubtedly has health benefits, and there is no doubt that certain diseases are less common here than in dirtier countries. But the practices also have some negative effects on health. Besides the fact that diseases acquired early in life can actually act as a sort of natural vaccination, preventing less serious forms of the disease later in life, as mentioned in the chapter on French medicine, too much cleaning zeal can directly cause medical problems. A large percentage of outer ear infections can be traced to cleaning the ears with cotton applicators, and vaginal ulcers have been linked to women's wearing of tampons between their menstrual periods to eliminate *all* discharge. Hysterectomies are performed because women don't like to put up with the supposed uncleanliness of their menstrual periods, and newborn boys circumcised for "hygienic" reasons.

Dr. Robert E. Hodges, a professor of internal medicine and chief of the section of nutrition in the school of medicine at the University of California at Davis suggests that "at least part of the inadequacy of the American diet can be attributed to our excessive concern over cleanliness. Our vegetables and fruits are thoroughly washed and peeled. Food is cooked in stainless steel, porcelainized or Teflon-coated pans, and our water supply passed through plastic or copper pipes. Much of the former opportunity for contamination of our food with iron and other essential minerals has been lost." And when you become anemic from iron deficiency, points out Dr. Paul Saltman of the University of California at San Diego, "your resistance to infection goes way, way down. People who are anemic are far more prone to infectious diseases, colds, viruses, bacterial infections and such."

Diseases that aren't explained by microbes are often explained in terms of other external agents, for example, foods, allergens, and carcinogens. Indeed, the banning of substances such as saccharin often causes great amusement in Europe. (The French found it odd that saccharin was banned for its supposedly carcinogenic properties, which they considered unproven: in France it is banned except in wartime for a more gastronomic reason: it is an "artificial" substance.)

Once a substance is branded as "bad," all complexities about whether it might be good for some people, or good in small quantities, vanish. Pregnant women, and even women trying to become pregnant, are told to avoid all alcohol, even though most studies have shown that drinking up to two glasses of wine a day throughout pregnancy does not increase the risk of harm to the fetus. New York City has legislated that all restaurants and bars post signs warning pregnant women that alcohol can cause birth defects, giving the impression that alcohol is some kind of nutritional thalidomide that can harm the fetus no matter how small the dose.

Salt, which causes blood pressure to rise in some people, but not everyone, was branded as "killer salt," bad for everyone, on the rationale that it would be easier to get people who were sensitive to salt to cut down if everyone cut down. Many people seemed to forget that in fact some salt is necessary to life, and a number of infants were severely harmed when an infant-food maker left all salt out of its formula, at least partly because it was trying to satisfy the demand of parents for lower-salt diets. Similarly, pregnant women were advised to reduce salt until it was realized that in fact they had fewer complications if they ate as much salt as they wanted. The egg was a similar scapegoat. The Welsh Dr. Archibald Cochrane recalls his American house-guest who asked him, shocked, "You mean you eat a whole egg for breakfast?" English doctors seem more likely than American ones to point out that some cholesterol may be good for you and that the high rate of stroke dropped in Japan at the same time they started eating more cholesterol. Americans, in fact, seem to want to be told that they should not eat certain substances: Dr. Pickering says that when the hypertension unit at New York Hospital does not tell people with high blood pressure that they should reduce their salt, many of the patients don't feel they are doing enough.

This preference for treating disease by exclusion (leaving or taking something out) rather than by inclusion (adding something, for example to the diet) has deep American roots. In the nineteenth century, wrote the historian Warner, not only were American diseases considered stronger than European diseases, but the American constitution was also considered energetic. This dictated that while enfeebled Europeans usually required therapeutic elevation when sick, Americans required repletion to drain off excess energy. Perhaps the exclusion of salt from the diet can be seen as the modern-day equivalent of bloodlet-

ting, since it, too, reduces blood volume, albeit in a less debili-
tating way.

The preference for taking something out, rather than adding
something, may also explain why America has been extremely
successful (many would say too successful) in regulating what
drugs can be used, yet much less so in regulating surgery. Surgery accords too much with our national mentality that if something is troublesome it should simply be removed. "Cut it out"
in fact is used as an all-purpose expression.

That peculiarly American institution, the checkup, was first called
the "health audit" shortly after World War I, when the prein-
duction physicals of soldiers-to-be showed them to be in de-
plorable health. The business metaphor soon changed to a
mechanical one, perhaps concurrent with the growing popularity of the automobile. According to Stanley Joel Reiser's *Medicine and the Reign of Technology*, "During the 1920s many
campaigns were launched to promote this idea, which used
slogans such as 'Have a health examination on your birthday,'
and posters carrying such messages as 'Your body is a wonderful
machine. You own and operate it. You can't buy new lungs
and heart when your own are worn out. Let a doctor overhaul
you once a year,' " seemingly ignoring the contradiction that if
the body *were* a machine, it should be possible to buy new lungs
and heart.

Body as car apparently caught the American imagination,
and the metaphor was embellished. "Think of your body as a
superautomobile," reads a typical American how-to book, *How
to Live Cheap But Good*. "If you don't drive it too fast for too
long, and if you feed it the right fuel, give it periodic checkups,
and maybe wash it occasionally, you'll prevent major rumblings
or at least treat them before they climax in a transmission."

And in a recent letter to *The New York Times Magazine*: "If he
would stop thinking of his body as a 1947 Chevy and start
taking care of the 1937 Rolls, he would be in better shape. My
model is 1923, and it has had the necessary periodontal work;

the varicose veins have been stripped; the windshields have been replaced with bifocal models and upgraded. The paint is still the original, but the soft top has thinned, revealing the excellent hard top below." When a Frenchman goes on vacation, it is to rest, or to "change ideas." An American goes to "recharge his batteries."

Perhaps it was an extreme application of the machine (and business) metaphor that prompted the U.S. Labor Department to announce in December 1985 that it was drafting a proposal whereby civilian federal employees would not be compensated for losing certain body parts such as sex organs, breasts, kidneys, or lungs in the line of duty. Officials believed, according to press reports at the time, that these organs were not necessary for the production of income. The department would continue to compensate workers for the loss of other body parts such as legs, arms, hands, or fingers.

The popularity of the idea of body as machine may explain why coronary bypass surgery caught on very quickly in the United States, reaching rates up to twenty-eight times that in some European countries. While the frequency with which the operation is performed has subsided somewhat in this country, and increased somewhat in Europe, the rate of the operation is still severalfold higher than in most European countries. The rationale of the operation is based on a very mechanical notion of the heart—that when an artery that brings blood to the heart is blocked, that artery must be bypassed with one that isn't blocked. Doctors in fact often speak of the day when there will be a sort of therapeutic Drāno—thus completing the machine image with a plumbing one.

When the operation was eventually studied in a controlled trial it was found that while certain persons (those with disease in the left main artery and perhaps those with disease in the three main coronary arteries) definitely enjoyed a longer life following bypass, for most patients the operation had no effect on how long they lived, although it did improve their quality of life by reducing symptoms of angina.

A member of a panel who evaluated the operation for the National Institutes of Health explained the popularity of the machine-operation in terms of the frontier mentality: that the operation was successful because patients often "want to be seen as men, as husbands, as providers, and they are willing to risk their lives at the time of the operation so as not to change their life-styles."

In theory, the large proportion of psychiatrists in America—over three times that of England, for example—would seem to contradict the man-as-machine image, but in fact, many psychiatrists seem to see the *mind* as a machine or even as plumbing. Dr. Michael O'Donnell, a former editor of *World Medicine* in London, says that an expatriate British psychiatrist, Dr. Bruce Sloame, chairman of the department of psychiatry at the University of Southern California, introduced him to the "Saniflush" concept of psychiatry in America. "This depends on people believing they all have it within themselves to achieve greatness—indeed to become president—if only some therapist could flush out those inhibitions and complexes that get in the way and hold them back."

In Janet Malcolm's book *Psychoanalysis: The Impossible Profession*, her analyst says, "Analysis isn't intellectual. It isn't moral. It isn't educational. It's an operation. It rearranges things inside the mind the way surgery rearranges things inside the body—even the way an automobile mechanic rearranges things under the hood of the car."

And in another of Ms. Malcolm's books, her controversial *In the Freud Archives*, she quotes Dr. Jeffrey Moussaief Masson as saying that his exposure of Freud's dishonesty about the seduction theory would have this effect: "They would have to recall every patient since 1901. It would be like the Pinto."

This approach, of course, was probably inevitable as psychiatrists had to justify their activities to a country that was not given to soul searching. Descartes had divided the body and the mind, but, being French, gave a great deal of priority to the mind and in fact constructed the entire world starting with a thought. Americans separate the mind and the body, but tend to prefer the body, justifying the mind in bodily terms. One study of psychiatric teaching showed psychiatrists telling medical students that "the mental status evaluation is just like the workup for a heart murmur . . . don't cardiologists teach you to ausculate the heart sounds systematically?"

Bruno Bettelheim in his book *Freud and Man's Soul* points out how when Freud's teachings were brought to the United States they lost much of the spiritual quality that Freud had given them. Freud often wrote about the soul, he said, but nobody who reads him in English could guess this, because nearly all his many references to the soul and to matters pertaining to the soul were excised in translation.

Freud instead was seen by English-language readers as "scientific." "Instead of instilling a deep feeling for what is most human in all of us, the translations attempt to lure the reader into developing a 'scientific' attitude toward man and his actions, a 'scientific' understanding of the unconscious and how it conditions much of our behavior."

Bettelheim says that "In the United States, of course, 'the cure of mental illness' has been seen as the main task of psychoanalysis, just as the curing of bodily illness is that of medicine. It is expected that anyone undergoing psychoanalysis will achieve tangible results—the kind of results the physician achieves for the body—rather than a deeper understanding of himself and greater control of his life."

This denial of the soul, or indeed even of the less mystical emotions, has taken its toll, too, on American medicine. Anything that cannot fit into the machine model of the body, or be quantified, is often denied not only quantification but even existence. As one doctor said of child-bearing centers: "We don't believe in taking an added risk in order to satisfy an emotional need. It's an indulgence."

The belief in the body as plumbing, coupled with the can-do approach, may be responsible for the fact that doctors in America, more than elsewhere in the world, try aggressively to keep terminally ill patients and even brain-dead patients alive on machines, often against their wishes and those of their families while at the same time neglecting the needs of the chronically ill and often the emotional needs of the acutely ill. It probably also explains the largely uncritical acclaim given to the artificial heart. Barney Clark became an American hero—or victim, if you will—because he was seen as a pioneer on the frontiers of medicine submitting to an extremely aggressive treatment based on a machine model of the human heart.

When reporters asked of the artificial heart whether the heart, the symbol of love, site of life, habitat of the soul, could be replaced by a simple mechanical pump, the director of the hospital's Division of Artificial Organs replied: "It's true that we may have palpitations, a rapid heart beat when we are in love, but this is secondary. If the owner of the artificial heart would find it pleasant to have these sensations, he can turn up the rate of the pump."

The artificial hearts failed, in the end, because they, unlike the human heart, were unable to adjust to the demands of the body and perhaps of the emotions. One day they may succeed, but for the moment the lesson remains: The heart may be just a pump, but it is a more sophisticated pump than human beings can yet mass produce.

Terminally ill patients being kept alive against their wishes, and perhaps even those who consent, such as Clark, may be seen as prisoners of the metaphors we use both in life and in medicine. But the metaphors, as we have seen, differ from culture to culture, and a broader look at those used elsewhere might show us that our choices are richer and more varied than we had imagined.

Such a look elsewhere might also demonstrate that our medicine is not the inevitable result of medical progress but of choices—conscious or not—that arise from our own cultural biases. Perhaps, if we come to know these biases better, our choices will reflect less the memory of a frontier past and more our needs as inhabitants of a complex modern society.

Plus Ça Change . . .

In October 1987, I was discussing the contents of this book with a French professor of medicine. One of his critiques was typically French: that I had not developed my topic theoretically. Another was typically medical: that medicine changes rapidly and that some of the treatments dealt with in this book were out of date. As an example he cited the treatment of breast cancer. No American doctor would take off a woman's breast now that science has shown that breast cancer is just as effectively treated by removing only part of the breast, he argued: such a doctor would certainly be sued by litigious American women. The very next day Nancy Reagan entered the hospital for a modified radical mastectomy: a treatment slightly less aggressive than the traditional Halsted radical mastectomy, but still more aggressive than the simple mastectomy favored in England and the less mutilating treatments favored in France.

A few weeks later I came upon an article dealing with the new drug treatments aimed at lowering cholesterol. In the article, a Canadian doctor alleged that while in England doctors start treating patients for high cholesterol only when a patient's blood cholesterol level reaches 300 milligrams per deciliter of cholesterol, in the United States treatment may begin at 225 milligrams, and some doctors are suggesting even lower levels.

New developments in medical science continue to be seen through cultural prisms; and while some of the treatments cited in this book may disappear as medical information is diffused throughout the world, those that most strongly reflect culture biases will persist in some form as long as those culture biases exist.

Can it be otherwise? No. The choice of diagnoses and treatments is *not* a science. While scientifically conducted studies can show us that a certain course of action or treatment can result in certain benefits and risks, the weighing of those benefits and risks will always be made on a cultural scale. How does the doctor of a cancer patient weigh the benefit of living a few more months against the risks (and unpleasantness) of feeling nauseated a good part of the time? How does the doctor of a patient with high blood pressure weigh the slightly reduced risk of heart attack and stroke against the impotence and other side effects many middle-aged men who are treated with drugs may suffer? How does one decide that, for a given patient, a little exposure to germs is preferable to a sanitized life-style? There is no easy answer, no mathematical formula that can factor risks and benefits and come up with a pat answer as to which treatment should be given and whether treatment should be given at all. In fact, only a patient is really competent to decide if there is a treatment of choice—for the patient.

Was it wrong for Nancy Reagan's doctors to have counseled her to have the mastectomy? No, not if they explained honestly what the likely consequences of each form of treatment were. There are reasons that a woman might make the choice Mrs. Reagan did: for example, a patient might favor traditional treatments, or be reluctant to undergo radiotherapy, or seek to avoid the worry that the cancer might come back in that breast. If those were, in fact, Nancy Reagan's priorities, then in this case the culture biases of the patient may well have accorded with those of her doctors. But it is wrong to say that the treatment she received is somehow "better" than other treatments. Perhaps better for her; probably not for many other women.

While medical ethicists and some enlightened doctors are beginning to see the large role value judgments play in medicine and realize that this implies a larger role for the patient in the making of medical decisions, most doctors, of course, continue to hide behind the screen of "scientific" medicine that somehow takes precedence over "unscientific" patient desires.

But we should not altogether blame doctors. As this book has attempted to show, while doctors may not realize it, they are often merely responding to the perceived or real demands of their patients. American medicine is aggressive partly because doctors are trained to be aggressive but also because many patients equate aggressive with better. Indeed, when I hear that someone has a reputation as a very good doctor I have come to expect someone who is aggressive and who favors radical surgery. But, particularly in countries like the United States, where it is easy to change doctors, patients have a good deal of power, if only they knew how to use it. When we as patients stop demanding aggressive, quick solutions to fix the machine, our doctors will gradually stop giving them.

Notes

Is Medicine International?

Page

15 "It is true . . .": Salvador de Madariaga, *Americans* (London: Oxford University Press, 1930).

16 This view became difficult: According to the 1986 *World Health Statistics Annual*, published by the World Health Organization (Geneva), in 1983 the life expectancy for U.S. men was 71 years and for U.S. women 78.3. The 1984 figures for England and Wales were men, 71.9; women, 77.9. The 1984 figures for France were men, 71.7; women, 80.1. The 1985 figures for West Germany were men, 71.6; women, 78.3. Infant mortality figures for the United States (1983) were 10.9 per 1,000 live births; the United Kingdom (1983) 10.0; France (1982) 9.4; and West Germany (1983) 10.2.

16 Documenting these different practices: *3ème Journée Nationale du K* (Nov. 30, 1982), Le Service National du Contrôle Médical, Caisse Nationale de l'Assurance Maladie des Travailleurs Salariés, Paris, 1985.

17 Even when comparative studies exist: W. A. Knaus et al., "A Comparison of Intensive Care in the U.S.A. and in France," *The Lancet*, Sept. 18, 1982, 642–46; L. L. Davitz, J. R. Davitz, and Y. Higuchi, "Cross-cultural Inferences of Physical Pain and Psychological Distress," *Nursing Times*, Apr. 14, 1977, 521–58; Apr. 21, 1977, 556–58. While the rate of D&C's has dropped sharply in recent years, in 1983 632,000 were performed, making it the third most common procedure performed in the United States. I. M. Rutkow, "Obstetric and Gynecologic Operations in the United States, 1979–1984," *Obstetrics and Gynecology* 67 (1986):755–59.

18 For the most part, I have tried to limit my inquiry: R. K. Schicke, "Socioeconomic Systems of Medicaments," *Social Science and Medicine* 10 (1976):277–81; P. U. Unschuld, "The Issue of Scientific and Alternative Medical Systems: A Comparison of East and West German Legislation," *Social Science and Medicine* 14B (1980):15–24.

20 My search for explanations: "Medical Personnel in the United Kingdom:

Analysis of Hospital Doctors by Specialty and Grade," Department of Health and Social Security, United Kingdom, 1980.

21 As Robert Damton wrote: Robert Damton, *The Great Cat Massacre and Other Episodes in French Cultural History* (New York: Basic Books, 1984), 4.

Cultural Bias in Medical Science

Page

23 "You will find . . .": M. N. G. Dukes, "Personal View," *British Medical Journal*, Sept. 1, 1973, 496.

23 "The literature shows . . .": Manfred Pflanz, "Problems and Methods in Cross-National Comparisons of Diagnoses and Diseases," in *Cross-National Sociomedical Research: Concepts, Methods, Practice*, eds. Manfred Pflanz and Elisabeth Schach (Stuttgart: Georg Thieme, 1976).

23 A French professor: T. A. Preston, *Coronary Artery Surgery: A Critical Review* (New York: Raven Press, 1977), 173.

24 Some of the most commonly prescribed drugs: Figures for drug use and common diagnoses come from Bernie O'Brien, *Patterns of European Diagnoses and Prescribing* (London: Office of Health Economics, 1984). Additional data on the high rate of cardiovascular prescribing in West Germany can be found in H. Freibal, "Arzneimittelverbrauch," *Deutsche Apotheker Zeitung* 15 (Apr. 15, 1982):815–18, and F. H. Gross, "Drug Utilization Data in Risk/Benefit Analyses of Drugs—Benefit Analysis," *Acta Medica Scandinavica Supplementa* 683 (1984):141–47.

Examples of ten- to twenty-fold differences in drug doses include the French use of bismuth as a laxative, where doses of 20 grams were used in contrast to half a gram to one gram in West Germany (personal communication from Dr. Karl Kimbel of the German Drug Commission in Cologne); and antacid use for ulcers in the United States, where 30 milliliters are given several times a day, in contrast to the lower European dose of 10 milliliters whenever the patient needs it (Faizallah et al., "Is There a Place in the United Kingdom for Intensive Antacid Treatment for Chronic Peptic Ulceration?" *British Medical Journal* 289 (1984): 869–71.

Suppository data come from Charles Lenoir and Simone Sandier, *La Consommation pharmaceutique en France et aux U.S.A.* (Paris: CREDOC, 1976), 95.

Comparison of surgery rates between the United Kingdom and the United States comes from: R. J. C. Pearson et al., "Hospital Caseloads in Liverpool, New England and Uppsala," *The Lancet*, Sept. 7, 1968, 559–66; J. P. Bunker, "Surgical Manpower: A Comparison of Operations and Surgeons in the United States and in England and Wales," *New England Journal of Medicine* 282 (1970):135–44; Klim McPherson et al., "Regional Variations in the Use of Common Surgical Procedures: Within and Between England and Wales, Canada and the United States of America," *Social Science and Medicine* 15A (1981):273–88; E. Vayda, W. R. Mindell, and I. M. Rutkow, "A Decade of Surgery in Canada, England and Wales and the United States," *Archives of Surgery* 117 (1982):846–53; Sigrid Lichtner and Manfred Pflanz, "Appendectomy in the Federal Republic of Germany: Epidemiology and Medical Care Patterns," *Medical Care* 9, no. 4 (July–Aug. 1971), 311–30; Preston, *Coronary Artery Surgery.*

25 The same clinical signs: R. E. Kendell, "Psychiatric Diagnosis in Britain and the United States," *British Journal of Psychiatry Special Publication* 9 (1975):453–61; Pierre Pichot, "The Diagnosis and Classification of Mental Disorders in French-Speaking Countries: Background, Current Views and Comparison with Other Nomenclature", *Psychological Medicine* 12 (1982): 475–92. Dr. Federico Allodi, a Toronto psychiatrist, claims that within five years of arriving in Canada, young Latin American women will likely have lost several organs though polysurgery because their doctors do not understand what their reported symptoms mean. Martin Stuart-Harle, "Transcultural Medicine: The Average G.P. Isn't Equipped to Deal with It," *The Medical Post,* June 12, 1984, 56–57.

25 Blood pressure considered treatably high: The German *Rote Liste* (1984), Bundesverband der Pharmazeutischen Industrie e.V., Aulendorf. W. Brüggemann, *Kneipp Vademecum Pro Medico* (Würzburg: Sebastian Kneipp Naturmittel Verlag, 1980).

25 The differences are most marked: Dukes, "Personal View"; "The Accuracy and Comparability of Death Statistics," *WHO Chronicle* 21 (1967): 7–17; Constance Percy and A. Dolman, "Comparison of the Coding of Death Certificates Related to Cancer in Seven Countries," *Public Health Reports* 93, no. 4 (1978):335–50.

26 A psychiatric assessment: T. W. Harding and H. Adserballe, "Assessments of Dangerousness: Observations in Six Countries: A Summary of Results from a WHO Coordinated Study," *International Journal of Law and Psychiatry* 6 (1983):391–98.

26 Already, a difference emerges: L. S. Linn et al., "Differences in the Numbers and Costs of Tests Ordered by Internists, Family Physicians, and Psychiatrists," *Inquiry* 21 (Fall 1984):266–75; Jay Noren et al., "Ambulatory Medical Care: A Comparison of Internists and Family-General Practitioners," *New England Journal of Medicine* 302 (1980):11–16; Thomas Hill, "Doctors Differ on Curing Their Ills," *The Medical Post,* Sept. 11, 1979; S. J. Wroe et al., "Differences Between Neurological and Neurosurgical Approaches in the Management of Malignant Brain Tumours," *British Medical Journal* 293 (1986):1015–18; Joseph B. Kirsner, "Current Medical and Surgical Opinions on Important Therapeutic Issues in Inflammatory Bowel Disease," *American Journal of Surgery* 140 (1980):391–95.

26 The physician faced with a tired patient: David Mechanic, "Some Comparisons Between the Work of Primary Care Physicians in the United

States and England and Wales," *Medical Care* 10 (Sept.–Oct. 1972):402–20; G. N. Marsh, R. B. Wallace, and J. Whewell, "Anglo-American Contrasts in General Practice," *British Medical Journal*, May 29, 1976, 1321–25; G. E. Linhardt, Jr., Robert Moore, and J. L. Hill, "Comparison of Health Care Delivery in Britain and the United States," *Maryland State Medical Journal*, July 1982, 41–45.

27 But for the time being let us accept: There are numerous ways that culture bias can influence the way clinical trials are conducted, or whether they are conducted at all. A letter by John M. Goldring, for example, in *The Lancet*, Mar. 27, 1982, 745, claims that obstetricians in the United States refused to participate in a trial of home births versus birthing-center births and midwife- versus obstetrician-attended births and that the reason for their resistance was that they were afraid to face the economic consequences had the trial shown they weren't really necessary. Other discussions about bias in clinical trials can be found in D. L. Sackett and M. Gent, "Controversy in Counting and Attributing Events in Clinical Trials," *New England Journal of Medicine* 301 (1979):1410–12; Geoffrey Rose and D. J. P. Barker, "Aetiology of Disease—Selection of Controls," *British Medical Journal* 2 (1978):1616–17; Archibald Cochrane, *Effectiveness and Efficiency* (Nuffield Provincial Hospitals Trust, 1971).

28 In the chapters that follow, the reason RCTs: Methodology is only one reason an article may not be accepted; culture biases pertain here, too. For a discussion see J. S. Armstrong, "Research on Scientific Journals: Implications for Editors and Authors," *Journal of Forecasting* 1 (1982):83–104.

28 Dr. A. M. W. Porter: A. M. W. Porter, "Three Threats to Standards of Medical Practice," *The Lancet*, May 17, 1980, 1071–73; Hedley Atkins et al., "Treatment of Early Breast Cancer," *British Medical Journal*, May 20, 1972, 423–29.

28 English and Americans are constantly rediscovering: Marcel-Francis Kahn, "Letter: Vertebral Osteomyelitis and Bacterial Endocarditis," *Arthritis and Rheumatism* 25 (1982):600.

29 Doctors claim: "Beyond Calais," *British Medical Journal*, Sept. 11, 1976, 606; J. A. Farfor and J. P. Benhamou, "French-English Medical Glossary:1–5," *The Lancet*, Oct. 6 to Nov. 3, 1973, 788–89, 840, 901–2, 959, 1018–19.

29 A similar situation prevails: Pierre Pichot, "The Diagnosis and Classification of Mental Disorders in French-Speaking Countries: Background, Current Views and Comparison with Other Nomenclatures," *Psychological Medicine* 12 (1982):475–92.

30 Even if the science is understood: E. M. Glaser, "Letter: Acceptable and Unacceptable Risks," *British Medical Journal*, Oct. 15, 1977, 1028–29.

30 If such very subjective conclusions: C. B. Begg and P. P. Carbone, "Clin-

ical Trials and Drug Toxicity in the Elderly: The Experience of the Eastern Cooperative Oncology Group," *Cancer* 52 (1983):1986–92.

31 In fact, the American authors: "Minerva," "Views," *British Medical Journal* 288 (1984):153.

31 If a study fits: For more information on how some studies are accepted and others rejected, see D. M. Kessner, "Diffusion of New Medical Information," *American Journal of Public Health* 71 (1981):367–68. For the specific case of how studies showing that shaving of the pubic hair of pregnant women about to deliver was not necessary were rejected, see R. Johnston and R. S. Sidall, "Is the Usual Method of Preparing Patients for Delivery Beneficial or Necessary?" *American Journal of Obstetrics and Gynecology* 4 (1922):645–50; H. I. Kantor et al., "Value of Shaving the Pudendal-Perineal Area in Delivery Preparation," *Obstetrics and Gynecology* 25 (1965):509–12; C. S. Mahan and S. McKay, "Preps and Enemas—Keep or Discard?" *Contemporary Ob/Gyn*, Nov. 1983, 241–48. The paper showing the efficacy of horse-chestnut extract is H. Bisler et al., "Wirkung von Rosskastaniensamenextrakt auf die transkapilläre Filtration bein Chronischer Venöser Insuffizienz" ("Effect of horse-chestnut seed extract on transcapillary filtration in chronic venous insufficiency"), *Deutsche Medizinische Wochenshrift* 111 (1986):1321–29.

32 In general, doctors in all countries: Umberto Veronesi, at a symposium on cancer research in Venice, quoted in *Medical Month*, Dec. 1983, 16.

32 In the United States: Preston, *Coronary Artery Surgery*; J. E. Brody, "Obstetric Panel Says Caesarean Deliveries Needn't Be Repeated," *The New York Times*, Feb. 25, 1982. In spite of the 1982 guidelines of the American College of Obstetricians and Gynecologists, in 1985, 93.4 percent of women who had previously delivered by cesarean were again given cesareans. P. J. Placek, S. M. Taffel, and M. Moien, "Letter: Cesarean Rate Increases in 1985," *American Journal of Public Health* 77 (1987):241–42.

32 It is, of course, easier for doctors to reject: L. K. Altman, "New Bacterium Linked to Painful Stomach Ills, *The New York Times*, July 31, 1984, C1.

33 Rejection of study results: B. Velimirovic, "Editorial: Do We Still Need International Health Regulations?" *Journal of Infectious Diseases* 133 (1976):478–82.

33 The widespread ignorance: According to the *Demographic Yearbook 1980* (New York: United Nations, 1982), the 1978 death rate for ischemic heart disease in the United States is 294.3 (per 100,000 population, including men and women); for West Germany, the figure was 230.8; for the United Kingdom, 378.6; for France, 95.2. Deaths from other forms of heart disease were 29.1 in the United States; 98.1 in West Germany; 33.7 in the United Kingdom; and 95.2 in France. If the two figures are added together, they become 323.4 in the United States; 328.9 in West

Germany, 412.3 in the United Kingdom; and 190.4 in France. See also B. Junge, "Decline in Mortality in Japan, USA and the Federal Republic of Germany—the Contribution of the Specific Causes of Death," *Klinische Wochenschrift* 63 (1985):793–801.

34 Second, the different ways: Sir Derrick Dunlop and R. S. Inch, "Variations in Pharmaceutical and Medical Practice in Europe," *British Medical Journal* 1972 (3):749–52; Dr. Claudine Escoffier-Lambiotte, "Le Bismuth est-il devenu une substance vénéneuse?" *Le Monde*, Mar. 19, 1975, 9; Nicolas Beau, "Les accidents liés au bismuth n'ont pas d'explications scientifiques satisfaisantes," *Le Monde*, July 12, 1978; P. Shenon, "Dispute over Intent in Drug Case Divided F.D.A. and Justice Department," *The New York Times*, Sept. 19, 1985, A1.

France

Page

35 "There's no money . . .": "Cyclosporine A Used to Stop AIDS Evolution," *The Medical Post*, Jan. 7, 1986, 42.

"I don't act": "Elle Talks to Men," *International Elle*, Spring/Summer 1984.

36 Except, as I learned during those days in Strasbourg: Geoffrey Keynes, for example, a surgeon and brother of the economist John Maynard Keynes, was publicly advocating conservative treatment of breast cancer from 1929 onward. See Geoffrey Keynes, *The Gates of Memory* (Oxford: Oxford University Press, 1981), chap. 17; Hedley Atkins et al., "Treatment of Early Breast Cancer: A Report after Ten Years of a Clinical Trial," *British Medical Journal*, May 20, 1972, 423–29.

37 The late Spanish diplomat: Salvador de Madariaga, *Englishmen, Frenchmen and Spaniards* (New York: Hill and Wang, 1930); W. A. Glaser, *Health Insurance Bargaining: Foreign Lessons for Americans* (New York: Gardener Press, 1978), 50; U. E. Reinhardt and Simone Sandier, *Alternative Methods of Physician Remuneration and Their Effects on Physician Activity: An International Comparison* (Paris: CREDOC, 1983).

38 As a consequence of prices: J. C. Sournia, *Ces malades qu'on fabrique: la médecine gaspillée* (Paris: Editions du Seuil, 1977), 228.

38 "The quest for the touchstones . . .": Sanche de Gramont, *The French: Portrait of a People* (New York: G. P. Putnam's Sons, 1969), chap. 6. See also Phil Adephus, "I Think Therefore I Am . . . French," *Passion*, Summer 1985.

39 I was interviewing Monod: Claudine Escoffier-Lambiotte, "Victoire sur la grippe à l'Institut Pasteur," *Le Monde de la Médecine*, Feb. 7, 1973, 13. For the theory behind the Pasteur Institute flu vaccine, see S. Fazekas de St. Groth, "Evolution and Hierarchy of Influenza Viruses," *Archives of Environmental Health* 21 (1970):293–302.

39 More recently French AIDS researchers: L. K. Altman, "Search for an AIDS Drug Is Case History in Frustration," *The New York Times*, July 30, 1985, C1; editorial, "Cyclosporine Suppressing the Competitive Urge," *The Medical Post*, Nov. 12, 1985, 10.

40 When Professor W. W. Holland: W. W. Holland, "Prospects for Change in Health Services: Reflections on Visits to European Countries," *World Hospitals* 13, no. 3 (1977):113–17.

40 When French women started to complain: J.-M. Cheynier, "L'Accouchement sans douleur: avec ou sans anesthésie?" *Le Monde*, Aug. 6–7, 1975, 9. Other nationalities are also prone to Cartesian thinking, particularly when such thinking accords with their culture biases. As I try to show in the American chapter, Americans often insist that "aggressive therapy" should work even in the face of evidence that it doesn't and will find all kinds of ways to discount evidence even when it exists. What is perhaps more typically French is their love of "elegant" ideas. The role of the skin in immunity, for example, treated in the United States with headlines about "defenses," was dealt with in France as a "dialogue" between the dermis and the epidermis. P. Sengel, "Le dialogue du derme et de l'épiderme," *Le Monde de la Médecine*, Oct. 19, 1977, 19.

41 Some of the drugs popular in France: Bernie O'Brien, *Patterns of European Diagnoses and Prescribing* (London: Office of Health Economics, 1984); E. Bloomfield, R. C. Gilbertson, and J. L. Skinner, "French General Practice," *Journal of the Royal College of General Practitioners*, May 1979, 297–301.

41 the almost systematic prescription of lactobacillus: J. Rivière, "Quatre points de vue sur les laxatifs, les levures et les fortifiants: Le microbiologiste: une microflore intestinale," *Le Monde de la Médecine*, Mar. 2, 1977, 17–18.

42 The idea was good: "Acidophilus: Milky Bane to Cholesterol," *Science News*, Aug. 25, 1984, 18.

42 rather significant side effects: Personal communication from Dr. Daniel Rabreau, director of S.O.S. Hemorroïdes, Paris.

43 Cartesian thinking can explain: Pierre Pichot, *A Century of Psychiatry* (Paris: Editions Roger Dacosta, 1983), 75. For more information about French psychiatric diagnosis see P. J. Pichot, "The French Approach to Psychiatric Classification," *British Journal of Psychiatry* 144 (1984):113–18; P. Pichot, "The Diagnosis and Classification of Mental Disorders in French-Speaking Countries: Background, Current Views and Comparison with Other Nomenclatures," *Psychological Medicine* 12 (1982):475–92.

43 Through the mid-1960s: Sherry Turkle, *Psychoanalytic Politics: Freud's French Revolution* (New York: Basic Books, 1978).

44 "French thought does not take": de Madariaga, *Englishmen, Frenchmen and Spaniards*, 63; Adephus, "I Think Therefore I Am."

44 Dr. Ralph L. Thompson: Ralph L. Thompson, *Glimpses of Medical Europe* (Philadelphia and London, J. B. Lippincott, 1908). According to writers David Talbot and Larry Bush, when it became clear that LAV and HTLV-III were actually the same virus, Gallo and his colleagues rushed to explain that the French findings were not as detailed as his and were actually based upon his earlier research. "You can't simply publish a picture of a virus and some unspecified characterizations of it like the French did and have people accept it," sniffed Gallo's colleague Sam Broder, *Mother Jones*, Apr. 1985.

45 The French do "look well": M. von Cranach, "The Cross-National Comparability of Psychiatric Diagnoses," in *Cross-National Sociomedical Research: Concepts, Methods, Practice*, ed. Manfred Pflanz and Elisabeth Schach (Stuttgart: Georg Thieme, 1976).

45 Radiologists in all countries: According to figures from the DHSS, in 1980 there were 821 radiologists and 1,466 anesthetists in Great Britain. French figures come from *Eurohealth Handbook* (White Plains, N.Y.: Robert S. First, 1985).

46 One type of radiologic exam: H. Tristant and M. Benmussa, *Atlas de l'hystérosalpingographie* (Paris: Masson, 1981). In the introduction to this book, Professor Guy Ledoux-Lebard writes that in the doses used the hysterosalpingogram has never been shown to cause fetal malformations, seemingly ignorant of the fact that the side effects of X rays are generally cumulative, and can rarely be attributed to one examination or type of examination but are due to the total amount of radiation.

47 But the French may have the last word: P. J. Taylor, D. C. Cumming, and P. J. Hill, "Significance of Intrauterine Adhesions Detected Hysteroscopically in Eumenorrheic Infertile Women and Role of Antecedent Curettage in their Formation," *American Journal of Obstetrics and Gynecology* 139 (1981):239–42.

47 French fairy tales: I have been unable to determine just when French fairy tales began ending this way. When I mentioned the difference in endings to students of older French fairy tales, they seemed unaware that "lots of children" was a part of the ending, but modern French men and women all agreed that fairy tales ended not only with a "happily ever after" but "and had lots of children." I suspect that the ending may have been deliberately added as part of the natalist campaign. G. Suffert, "Natalité: le déclin français," *Le Point* 566 (July 25, 1983):31–36; "Low Birth Rate in Western Europe Means Big Social, Economic Changes Are Likely," *The Wall Street Journal*, Dec. 30, 1985, 16.

48 The concern about fertility: French infant mortality statistics can be found in *Eurohealth Handbook*; Federation CECOS, D. Schwartz, and M. J. Mayaux, "Female Fecundity as a Function of Age," *New England Journal of Medicine* 306 (1982):404–6; "Editorial: In Delay There Lies No Plenty," *The Lancet*, Mar. 20, 1982, 665. While the French normally have to pay a part of their doctor visits and prescription costs, women get completely free medical care for the last four months of their pregnancy; "Mme. Simone Veil a annoncé la gratuité des soins pendant les quatre derniers mois de la grossesse," *Le Monde*, Sept. 22, 1978.

48 Although French law: J. H. Soutoul and F. Pierre, "La stérilisation humaine volontaire," *Revue Française Gynécologie Obstétrique* 81 (1986):483–91. "L'Ordre des médecins engage la bataille contre la stérilisation volontaire," *Le Monde*, Jan. 12, 1978; S. Arlot et al., "Contraception chez la diabétique," *La Presse Médicale* 12 (1983):9–16.

49 Prior to getting a prescription: Claudine Escoffier-Lambiotte, "La Contraception vingt ans après: le coeur et les vaisseaux: de nécessaires précautions," *Le Monde de la Médecine*, Mar. 7, 1979, 13. Thérèse Lecomte and G. Bienenfeld, *Evolution de la morbidité déclarée, France 1970–1980* (Paris: CREDOC, 1983), 69.

49 In the 1970s: "Contraception 80: Tout ce que vous voulez savoir," *Marie-Claire*, Nov. 1980, 63; "Avantages et inconvénients du stérilet," *Le Monde*, Nov. 19, 1980, 20. American women were not really warned about the effect of the IUD on fertility until two studies published in 1985 found that IUDs doubled the risk of infertility. Janet Daling et al., "Primary Tubal Infertility in Relation to the Use of an Intrauterine Device," *New England Journal of Medicine* 312 (1985):937–41; D. W. Cramer et al., "Tubal Infertility and the Intrauterine Device," *New England Journal of Medicine* 312 (1985):941–47.

49 French women don't: "WFS [World Fertility Survey] Surveys Show That Western, Eastern Europe Differ Greatly in Use of Modern Contraceptives," *Family Planning Perspectives* 15 (Mar./Apr. 1983):82–84.

50 One French answer to contraception: Ibid.; L. R. Brown, "High- and Low-tech Birth Control," *Natural History*, Apr. 1985; de Gramont, *The French*, 406.

50 Another French practice: I. M. Rutkow, "Obstetric and Gynecologic Operations in the United States, 1979–1984," *Obstetrics and Gynecology* 67 (1986):755–59; Centers for Disease Control, "Surgical Sterilization Surveillance; Hysterectomy in Women Aged 15–44, 1976–78," Mar. 1981, 3. Comparisons between England and the United States show that England has half the U.S. rate of hysterectomy; and a survey of women in several European countries found that French rates were the lowest, lower than England's. P. A. van Keep, D. Wildemeersch, and P. Lehert, "Hysterectomy in Six European Countries," *Maturitas* 5 (1983):69–75.

51 Professor Netter: In 1980, the U.S. Center for Health Statistics showed 403,000 hysterectomies and 28,000 myomectomies performed.

52 these reasons were pooh-poohed: E. W. Munnell, "Total Hysterectomy," *American Journal of Obstetrics and Gynecology*, July 1947, 31–39.

52 the French may have been right: P. Kilkku, "Supravaginal Uterine Amputation vs. Hysterectomy: Effects on Coital Frequency and Dyspareunia," *Acta Obstetrica Gynecologica Scandinavica* 62 (1983):141–45; P. Kilkku et al., "Supravaginal Uterine Amputation vs. Hysterectomy: Effects on Libido and Orgasm," *Acta Obstetrica et Gynecologica Scandinavica* 62 (1983):147. See also L. Zussman et al., "Sexual Response After Hysterectomy-Oophorectomy: Recent Studies and Reconsideration of Psychogenesis," *American Journal of Obstetrics and Gynecology* 140 (Aug. 1, 1981), 725–29.

53 The importance of aesthetics: F. Plas, "La Rééducation postobstétricale," *Concours Médicaux* 104, no. 24 (June 12, 1982):3929–30; M. Harmanowicz et al., "Cancers du pénis: Technique d'amputation limité au glans," *La Presse Medicale*, Sept. 12, 1987, 1430–31.

54 The French focus on aesthetics: D. Beaumont, "Lifelike Hands Are Not for Everyone," *The Medical Post*, Nov. 3, 1981, 2.

54 Whether the French undergo: Freda Garmaise, "Bold Bosoms," *Village Voice*, Dec. 25, 1984, 43.

54 The figures from the United States: "Editorial: A Stone from Around the Neck," *The Medical Post*, Jan. 12, 1982, 12.

55 The French concern with thinness: The Utopian socialist Fourier, for example, set out a priori in great detail menus that would make community members look forward to the next meal and proposed replacing wars with international cooking contests. Jonathan Beecher, *Charles Fourier: The Visionary and His World* (Berkeley: University of California Press, 1986).

56 French eating and drinking habits: *Demographic Yearbook 1980* (New York: United Nations, 1982); Jean-Michel Warnet et al., "Relation Between Consumption of Alcohol and Fatty Acids Esterifying Serum Cholesterol in Healthy Men," *British Medical Journal* 290 (1985):1859–61; "Food and Mortality in France," *The Lancet*, July 16, 1977, 133.

57 French doctors examine the liver more: R. V. H. Jones, "A Week with a French Country Doctor," *Journal of the Royal College of General Practitioners* 24 (1974):689–93.

57 French patients and their doctors: Claude Béraud, *Le Foie des français* (Paris: Stock/Laurence Pernoud, 1983). I also came upon the fact that the Scottish doctor Thomas Percival introduced the use of cod liver oil into medical practice in 1782—after a trip to Paris! See P. Huard, "Les Echanges médicaux franco-anglais au XVIIIe siècle," *Clio Medica* 3 (1968):41–58.

58 The *crise de foie*: Lauren Julia Batta, "Les Mythes Médicaux Français: Alcoolisme, Thermalisme, et La Crise de Foie," thesis, Princeton University, 1986.

58 biliary dyskinesia: A. Gerolami, "Dyskinésies Biliaires," in Pierre Godeau, Serge Herson, and Jean-Charles Piette, *Traité de médecin*, 2nd ed. (Paris: Flammarion Médecine—Sciences, 1987), 1600–1601.

59 In 1970: D. Dhumeaux, "La Recherche en hépatologie: Le mythe de la 'crise de foie,' " *Cahiers médicaux* 2 (Oct. 11, 1976):337–38; Charles Lenoir and Simone Sandier, *La Consommation pharmaceutique en France et aux U.S.A.* (Paris: CREDOC, 1976), 90.

59 In 1976: Press conference held under the auspices of the Institut National de la Santé et de la Recherche Médicale, on June 3, 1976; Lecomte and Bienenfeld, *Evolution de la morbidité déclarée*, 73; O'Brien, *Patterns of European Diagnoses*, 17.

60 Nearly 7.5 percent of French drugs: Lenoir and Sandier, *Consommation pharmaceutique*, 95; F. M. Hull, "A Day with the Doctor: France," *Update*, Apr. 1, 1979. A negative aspect of suppositories is that they can lead to hemorrhoids. Jean Duhamel, "Les Hémorroïdes: un mal qu'il est possible de guérir, mais aussi d'éviter," *Le Monde*, Aug. 10, 1977, 10.

60 While a common anemia in England or America: Jacques Messerschmitt, *La Médecine contre la santé* (Paris: Editions Debard, 1982). Martin Shapiro and colleagues, investigating the diagnosis and treatment of low blood pressure in a Canadian community, found that one of the treatments being used was veal liver extract and vitamin B_{12}. M. F. Shapiro, H. Korda, and J. Robbins, "Diagnosis and Treatment of Low Blood Pressure in a Canadian Community," *Canadian Medical Association Journal* 126 (1982):918–20.

60 In 1980, a French drug, Selacryn: P. Shenon, "Dispute Over Intent in Drug Case Divided F.D.A. and Justice Dept.," *The New York Times*, Sept. 19, 1985, A1; "Man Sees What He Suspects," *British Medical Journal* 290 (1985):1654.

62 Focus on the *terrain* shapes French medicine: Lenoir and Sandier, *Consommation pharmaceutique*, 90; O'Brien, *Patterns of European Diagnoses*, 30.

62 Spasmophilia, a uniquely French diagnosis: Lecomte and Bienenfeld, *Evolution de la morbidité déclarée*, 69.

63 But what is spasmophilia?:For more about spasmophilia, see H.-P. Klotz, *Etre Spasmophile et bien-portant* (Paris: Presses de la Renaissance, 1982); J. Heim and B. Plouvier, "Pour (tenter d') en finir avec la spasmophilie," *Concours médicaux*, Nov. 20, 1982, 6483; R. Gérard et al., "Prolapsus valvulaire mitral et spasmophilie chez l'adulte," *Archives des Maladies du Coeur et des Vaisseaux* 72, no. 7 (1979):715–20; J. Gatau-Pelanchon et al., "Prolapsus mitral et spasmophilie chez l'enfant et l'adolescent," *Archives des Maladies du Coeur et des Vaisseaux* 72, no. 5 (1979), 449–53; Y. Numera et al., "Symptomatologie observée chez 162 malades classés comme spasmophile (Tétanie chronique idiopathique ou constitutionelle)," *Annales de Médecine interne* 129, no. 1 (Jan. 1979):9–15.

63 Spasmophilia probably corresponds most closely: T. F. Waites, "Hyperventilation—Chronic and Acute," *Archives of Internal Medicine* 138 (1978):1700–01; R. Liberthson et al., "The Prevalence of Mitral Valve Prolapse in Patients with Panic Disorders," *American Journal of Psychiatry* 143, no. 4 (1986):4, 511–15; L. D. Galland, S. M. Baker, and R. K. McLellan, "Letter: Irritable Bowel, Mitral Valve Prolapse, and Associated Conditions," *Journal of the American Medical Association* 254 (1985):358–59.

65 In the United States, it is rare: Nicolas Beau, "Huit malades sur cent ont recours à l'homéopathie," *Le Monde*, Apr. 23–24, 1978, 8; J. Lyall, "Attitudes to Medicine: France," *Self Health*, June 1984; George Dunea, "Counting Sheep and Eating Herbs," *British Medical Journal* 293 (1986):1019–20.

65 A 1984 *Guide pratique des médecines douces*: S. Tenenbaum, *Le Guide pratique des médecines douces* (Paris: Editions Retz, 1984).

66 In a 1976 CREDOC comparison: Lenoir and Sandier, *Consommation pharmaceutique*, 90; O'Brien, *Patterns of European Diagnoses*, 30. The belief in gentle treatment goes back a long way in French medicine. François Magendie (1783–1855), who taught Claude Bernard, was keenly skeptical about many kinds of accepted medical treatment; he felt that the less vigorously the patient was treated, the better; from J. Tarshis, *Claude Bernard, Father of Experimental Medicine* (New York: Dial Press, 1968).

66 The French preference: Gilles Bardelay, "Posologie du paracetamol, qui a raison?" *La Revue Prescrire*, Apr. 1987, 224–26.

66 A belief in the *terrain*: W. A. Knaus et al., "A Comparison of Intensive Care in the U.S.A. and in France," *The Lancet*, Sept. 18, 1982, 642–46.

66 Another consequence is more limited operations: C. Missirliu, "Le Prépuce de l'enfant," *Cercle d'études pédiatriques*, *Le Pédiatre* 8, no. 40 (1972):351–59.

67 One famous French surgeon: Howard W. Haggard, *Devils, Drugs and Doctors* (William Heinemann, 1929); Pierre Leulliette, "Au Nom de la loi," *Le Monde*, Oct. 10–11, 1976, 13; A. Corbin, *The Foul and the Fragrant: Odor and the French Social Imagination* (Cambridge, Mass.: Harvard University Press, 1986); "La Peau sans répit," *Le Monde*, Sept. 6, 1972, 13; H. Laskey, "A Shower of Arguments Against Being Squeaky Clean," *The Medical Post*, Apr. 21, 1987; Views, *British Medical Journal* 291 (1985):145.

68 For many years French dermatologists: When I was first told this, shortly after arriving in France in 1971, I found the idea quite strange. However, when I came back to the United States in the 1980s, I found that a few dermatologists were beginning to espouse it.

68 Many French doctors believe: R. Aron-Brunetière, *La Beauté et la médecine* (Paris: Stock, 1974); Nathalie Mont-Servan, "Les Shampooings passés au peigne fin," *Le Monde*, Jan. 7, 1978, 18. L. A. Schoen, ed., *A.M.A. Book of Skin and Hair Care* (New York: Avon, 1978).

68 Dry hair, oily hair, and acne: M. Hincky, J.-M. Hincky, and X. Fouillet, "Shampooings et séborrhées du cuir chevelu," *Le Concours Médical*, June 25, 1977, 4297–310.

68 too much cleanliness in restaurants: "Mises en Garde des autorités sanitaires contre des pâtés de foie," *Le Monde*, Oct. 21, 1977; Judith Miller, "In Périgord, a Furor over Foie Gras," *The New York Times*, Dec. 18, 1985. Miller reports that France requires *foie gras* imports to be "healthy, loyal and marketable."

69 A dirty life-style: Figures on antibody to hepatitis A come from Dr. Benhamou. A recent American study showed that students used to consuming raw milk had considerably more resistance to a Campylobacter infection than did students unused to consuming raw milk. After a retreat to an Oregon farm, 76 percent of those not used to drinking raw milk got sick, where none of the ten students used to consuming raw milk did. M. J. Blaser, E. Sazie, and L. P. Williams, Jr., "The Influence on Raw Milk–Associated Campylobacter Infection," *Journal of the American Medical Association* 257 (1987):43–46.

70 Still another aspect of *terrain*: "Sortie précoce de l'hôpital après l'accouchement: les femmes peu favorables," *Le Concours Médical*, Feb. 4, 1984, 353–54.

70 French sick leaves: Messerschmitt, *Médecine contre la santé*, 49.

71 The belief in rest: H. le Brigand, in *La Tuberculose—une victoire thérapeutique oui mais . . .* (Paris: Collection Prospective et Santé Publique Group 9, 1973), 20.

71 "The idea of the unhealthy character . . .": Turkle, *Psychoanalytic Politics*, 37.

71 One in every two hundred: Thérèse Lecomte, and P. Le Fur, *Les Médecins libéraux: Clientèle et prescription-enquête pilote* (Paris: CREDOC, 1982), 34; H. Bouchet, "Les 4ᵉ Thermalies," *La Presse Médicale* 14, no. 14 (Apr. 6, 1985):796; G. Ebrard, *Le Thermalisme en France: Situation actuelle et perspectives d'avenir* (Paris: La Documentation Française, 1981).

Germany

74 "He seems to value my mind . . .": J. W. von Goethe, *The Sorrows of Young Werther* (1774; reprint, New York: Signet, 1982).

74 "The heart is the key . . .": In L. A. Willoughby, *The Romantic Movement in Germany* (Oxford: Oxford University Press, 1930).

74 statistics on German drug use: H. Freibel, "Arzneimittelverbrauch," *Deutsche Apotheker Zeitung*, 15, no. 15 (Apr. 1982):815–18.

74 It's not because . . . : See note to page 135.

74 huge consumption of heart drugs: EVaS Study 1981/82, Zentral Institut für die Kassenärztliche Versorgung in der Bundesrepublik Deutschland, Köln, Federal Republic of Germany, in *Third International Conference on System Science in Health Care*, ed. W. van Eimeren, R. Engelbrecht, and Ch. D. Flagle, (Berlin: Springer-Verlag, 1984); Bernie O'Brien, *Patterns of European Diagnoses and Prescribing* (London: Office of Health Economics, 1984); J. R. Moehr and K. D. Haehn, *Verdenstudie* (Köln-Lövenich: Deutscher Artze-Verlag, 1977); J. Schaefer, "The Case Against Coronary Artery Surgery: A Paradigm for Studying the Nature of a So-called Scientific Controversy in the Field of Cardiology," *Metamedicine* 1 (1980):155–76.

75 The . . . movement known as romanticism: Willoughby, *The Romantic Movement*; Owsei Temkin, "German Concepts of Ontogeny and History Around 1800," in *The Double Face of Janus and Other Essays in the History of Medicine* (Baltimore: Johns Hopkins University Press, 1977).

75 The basic concepts of this philosophy: F. H. Garrison, "Editorial: The Romantic Episode in the History of German Medicine," *Bulletin of the New York Academy of Medicine* 7 (1931):841–64.

76 the German character: Maya Pines, "Unlearning Blind Obedience in German Schools," *Psychology Today*, May 1981.

77 The West German health care system: P. U. Unschuld, "The Issue of Structured Coexistence of Scientific and Alternative Medical Systems: A Comparison of East and West German Legislation," *Social Science and Medicine* 14B (1980):15–24.

78 While German drug laws: Ibid.; Tony Smith, "Limited Lists of Drugs: Lessons from Abroad," *British Medical Journal* 290 (1985):532–34.

78 Drugs also are frequently prescribed: "West Germany: An Overabundance of Drugs," *The Lancet*, Oct. 8, 1977, 756.

78 Perhaps because both fringe and high-tech medicine are accepted: There are 232 doctors for every 100,000 inhabitants in West Germany, 207 in the United States, 214 in France, and 154 in the United Kingdom. Yan Blanpain, Bjorn Lindgren, and Simone Sandier, *Comparisons internationales des systemes de santé* (Paris: Centre de Recherche d'Etude et de Documentation en Economie de la Santé, 1985); U. E. Reinhardt and Simone Sandier, *Alternative Methods of Physician Remuneration and Their Effects on Physician Activity: An International Comparison* (Paris: CREDOC, 1983); O'Brien, *Patterns of European Diagnoses.*

79 One study found: Moehr and Haehn, *Verdenstudie*, 75; Reinhardt and Sandier, *Alternative Methods*; F. M. Hull, "A Day with the Doctor: Germany," *Update*, Sept. 15, 1980, 607–12.

79 Patients seem unlikely: O'Brien, *Patterns of European Diagnoses*, 7; J. W. Tanner,"Prolonged Study Leave in Hamburg and Vienna," *Journal of the Royal College of General Practitioners* 27 (1977):436–37.

79 "Overdoctoring" is a danger here: Freibel, "Arzneimittelverbrauch"; O'Brien, *Patterns of European Diagnoses*; Franz Gross, "Drug Utilization Data in Risk/Benefit Analyses of Drugs—Benefit Analysis," *Acta Medica Scandinavica Supplementa* 683 (1984):141–47; B. Junge, "Decline in Mortality in Japan, USA, and the Federal Republic of Germany—the Contribution of the Specific Causes of Death," *Klinische Wochenschrift* 63 (1985):793–801.

80 The Germans knew better: Schaefer, "Case Against Coronary Artery Surgery."

81 The German concept of the heart: Junge, "Decline in Mortality."

81 The German way of looking at the heart: Schaefer, "Case Against Coronary Artery Surgery"; "Lapses of the Heart," *Hastings Center Report*, June 1986, 46; K. Lempke and H.-H. Klare, "Er Starb Zwei Jahre," *Stern*, Aug. 14, 1986, 114. The role of Germany in developing calcium channel blockers—drugs that act against spasm of the coronary artery—was acknowledged in a press conference given in New York on June 10, 1983, by Pfizer Pharmaceuticals.

81 But another reason: Moehr and Haehn, *Verdenstudie*, 108; O'Brien, *Patterns of European Diagnoses*; EVaS Study 1981/82, in *Third International Conference*, ed. van Eimeren, Englebrecht, and Flagle.

81 One of the first ways: German office-based doctors take an electrocardiogram in 2.9 percent of office visits (personal communication based on the EVaS Study from Dr. B.-P. Robra), similar to the 2.7 percent of U.S. office visits (Thomas McLemore, "1979 Summary, National Ambulatory Medical Care Survey," NCHS Advance Data Number 66, Mar. 2, 1981).

82 But since the West German patient: Ulrich Geissler, of the Research Institute of the Federation of Local Health Insurance Funds Association in Bonn, estimated that in 1979, 1,267,000 ECGs were performed in the Ruhr area of West Germany, which has a population of 5.2 million— in other words, one of every five Germans had an ECG in a year.

83 According to other observers: W. H. Helfand, "The United States and the International Pharmaceutical Market," *Journal of the American Pharmaceutical Association* 10 (1970):658–63; Moehr and Haehn, *Verdenstudie*, 108; R. Dreibholz et al., "Häufigkeit von Krankheitsbezeichnungen in fünf Allgemeinpraxen," *Allgemeinmedizin International* 1 (1974):21–25.

86 Low blood pressure . . . the "German disease": Moehr and Haehn, *Verdenstudie*, 108, shows that hypotension was the seventeenth most common diagnosis seen, about one-sixth as often as high blood pressure. EVaS Study 1981/82, in *Third International Conference*, ed. van Eimeren, Englebrecht, and Flagle. *Rote List* (1984), Bundesverband der Pharmazeutischen Industrie e.V., Aulendorf.

86 While low blood pressure was occasionally mentioned: J. M. Robbins, H. Korda, and M. F. Shapiro, "Treatment for a Nondisease: The Case of Low Blood Pressure," *Social Science and Medicine* 16 (1982):27–33; M. F. Shapiro, "Low Blood Pressure: An Extinct Diagnosis," *Canadian Medical Association Journal* 126 (1982):887–88.

88 Poor circulation . . . is blamed: Kurt Raab, "My Life with Rainer," *Village Voice*, May 3, 1983. The West Germans have even introduced a product to improve circulatory disorders—in dogs; "Making Rexy Sexy," *MD*, Nov. 1985, 28. They have also developed a diagnostic test for varicose veins, phlebitis, and other venous problems that works by directing infrared light beams through the skin and into the veins while the patient performs a series of exercises. Monica Shea, "What Your Patients Are Reading," *Medical Post*, Apr. 3, 1984, 38.

The predominance of circulatory disorders can be seen in the list of the twenty most common German diagnoses in O'Brien, *Patterns of European Diagnoses*; "other" myocardial insufficiency ranks first, hypertension third, varicose veins tenth ischemic cerebrovascular disease seventeenth. By contrast, of the twenty leading diagnoses in the United Kingdom, only hypertension and symptoms—cardiovascular and lymphatic system (in fifteenth place)—made the top twenty. In the EVaS Study, of the ten most frequent principal reasons for visits with general practitioners, vertigo-dizziness was in second place, shortness of breath in sixth, heart pain in seventh, leg symptoms in tenth.

89 Rudolf Virchow: Erwin H. Ackerknecht, *Rudolf Virchow: Doctor, Statesman, Anthropologist* (Madison: University of Wisconsin Press, 1953).

90 A 1980 book on Kneipp therapy: W. Brüggemann, *Kneipp Vademecum Pro Medico* (Würzburg: Sebastian Kneipp Naturmittel Verlag, 1980). For more information about Kneipp, see A. Schalle, *Die Kneipp Kur: Therapie, Anwendung, Erfolg* (München: Pawlak, n.d.); A. Moyle, in *A Visual Encyclopedia of Unconventional Medicine*, ed. A. Hill (New York: Crown, 1979).

92 The legacy of Virchow: Ackerknecht, *Virchow*; G. A. Silver, "Virchow, the Heroic Model in Medicine: Health Policy by Accolade," *American Journal of Public Health* 77 (1987):82–88.

93 That West German doctors still: O'Brien, *Patterns of European Diagnoses*, 31; Freibel, "Arzneimittelverbrauch."

94 While there may be: According to Dr. Dennis Maki, head of the infectious disease section at the University of Wisconsin school of medicine, much of the epidemic in hospital-acquired infections in the United States can be traced to an overzealous use of beta lactam antibiotics such as the cephalosporins over the last ten years. T. Sellers, "Prophylactic Antibiotics 'Overused' in Surgery," *The Medical Post*, Aug. 19, 1986, 68.

94 The relative importance given . . . to "inner" causes: A. Bloomfield, "Origin of the Term 'Internal Medicine,' " *Journal of the American Medical Association* 168 (1959):1628; R. A. Hahn, "Treat the Patient, Not the Lab: Internal Medicine and the Concept of 'Person,' " *Culture, Medicine and Psychiatry* 6:219–36.

94 German psychiatry has . . . : J. Marshall Townsend, "Cultural Conceptions and the Role of the Psychiatrist in Germany and America," *International Journal of Social Psychiatry* 24 (1978):250–58; G. Ammon, "Germany: Psychiatry," in *International Encyclopedia of Psychiatry, Psychology, Psychoanalysis and Neurology* (New York: Aesculapius Publishers [Van Nostrand Reinhold Company], 1977).

96 The unacceptability of psychiatry: O'Brien, *Patterns of European Diagnoses*.

96 The medical use of spas: H. Bouchet, "Les 4ᵉ Thermalies," *La Presse médicale* 14, no. 14 (Apr. 6, 1985):796; R. K. Schicke, "Socio-Economic Systems of Medicaments," *Social Science and Medicine* 10 (1976):277–81.

97 About one-fifth of German M.D.'s: Unschuld, "Structured Coexistence."

97 Steiner, like many German philosophers: J. A. Dyson and C. Hollmann, "Anthroposophical Medicine," in *A Visual Encyclopedia of Unconventional Medicine* (New York: Crown, 1979).

98 Steiner's system also uses: "Homeopathic Remedies," *Consumer Reports*, Jan. 1987, 60–62; David T. Reilly et al., "Is Homeopathy a Placebo Response?" *The Lancet*, Oct. 18, 1986, 881–85; R. G. Gibson et al., "Homeopathic Therapy in Rheumatoid Arthritis: Evaluation by Double Blind Clinical Therapeutic Trial," *British Journal of Clinical Pharmacology* 1980, 9 (1980):453–59. See also Andrew Weil, *Health and Healing* (Boston: Houghton Mifflin, 1983).

99 Exactly how contact with homeopathy: M. V. Singer et al., "Low Concentrations of Ethanol Stimulate Gastric Acid Secretion Independent of Gastrin Release in Humans," *Gastroenterology* 86 (1985):1254.

England

Page

101 The most striking characteristic of British medicine: U. E. Reinhardt and Simone Sandier, *Alternative Methods of Physician Remuneration and Their Effects on Physician Activity: An International Comparison* (Paris: CREDOC, 1983); G. N. Marsh, R. B. Wallace, and J. Whewell, "Anglo-American Contrasts in General Practice," *British Medical Journal*, May 29, 1976, 1321–25; David Mechanic, "General Medical Practice: Some Comparisons Between the Work of Primary Care Physicians in the United States and England and Wales," *Medical Care* 10 (1972):402–20; A. M. W. Porter and J. M. T. Porter, "Anglo-French Contrasts in Medical Practice," *British Medical Journal*, Apr. 26, 1980, 1109–12; G. Worrall, "Our Way: Long Hours, Few Vacations, Poor Records," *The Medical Post*, Apr. 3, 1984, 54; F. M. Hull, "International Sore Throats," *Journal of the Royal College of General Practitioners* 31 (1981):45–48.

102 The British patient receives: Henry J. Aaron and William B. Schwartz, *The Painful Prescription* (Washington, D.C.: Brookings Institute, 1984); "Spotty Shadows on Chest X-ray Pose Diagnostic Dilemma for Physicians," *The Medical Post*, May 23, 1978.

102 British doctors prescribe fewer drugs: Bernie O'Brien, *Patterns of European Diagnoses and Prescribing* (London: Office of Health Economics, 1984); Sir Derrick Dunlop and R. S. Inch, "Variations in Pharmaceutical and Medical Practice in Europe," *British Medical Journal* 3 (1972):749–52; Editorial, "Vasodilators in Senile Dementia," *British Medical Journal*, Sept. 1, 1979, 511–12; H. Freibel, "Arzneimittelverbrauch," *Deutsche Apotheker Zeitung* 15, no. 15 (Apr. 1982):815–18; Aaron and Schwartz, *The Painful Prescription*; J. P. Horder and John Hunt, "A French View of English General Practice," *Journal of the Royal College of General Practitioners* 25 (1975):365–67; C. Francome and P. J. Huntingford, "Births by Caesarean Section in the United States of America and in Britain," *Journal of*

Biosocial Science 12 (1980):353–62; R. J. C. Pearson et al., "Hospital Caseloads in Liverpool, New England, and Uppsala," *The Lancet*, Sept. 7, 1968, 559–66; T. B. Hargreave, "Radical Cystectomy," *British Medical Journal* 290 (1985):338–39. British doctors are also less likely to immunize for measles. N. D. Noah, "Measles Eradication Policies," *British Medical Journal* 284 (1982):997–98.

103 High-technology medicine: R. A. Sells, S. MacPherson, and J. R. Salaman, "Assessment of Resources for Renal Transplantation in the United Kingdom," *The Lancet*, July 27, 1985, 195–97; "Editorial: Death by a Thousand Cuts," *British Medical Journal* 285 (1982):1–2. The reason why the patient in the coronary care unit had dark skin was pointed out by one of the museum staff.

103 Even vitamin requirements are smaller: "Round Table on Comparison of Dietary Recommendations in Different European Countries," *Nutrition and Metabolism* 21 (1976):223. A U.S. panel has recommended that the U.S. recommendation for vitamin C be reduced, bringing it more into line with the British recommendation. An expert British committee in 1983 recommended that the risk of overweight not be exaggerated in relation to the risk of continuing to smoke, made no recommendation about lowering cholesterol intake, and voiced the recommendation about salt intake mildly as, "It would be desirable if salt intakes on average fell by 3 gram per head per day." W. P. T. James et al., "A Discussion Paper on Proposals for Nutritional Guidelines for Health Education in Britain," prepared for the National Advisory Committee on Nutrition Education (London: Health Education Council, 1983).

103 Very few screening exams: Bev Daily, "The Way You Say It," *MD*, June 1986, 49ff. "Editorial: Management of Abnormal Cervical Smears," *British Medical Journal*, May 24, 1980, 1239–40. In 1987, the British government announced it was setting up a breast-cancer screening program, with screening of women between the ages of 50 and 64 once every three years. There were no plans to screen women under 50. "Breast Cancer Screening for Brits. 50–64," *The Medical Post*, Apr. 7, 1987; I. Goldman, "Lax Cancer Screening Attitudes Have to Change," *The Medical Post*, May 14, 1985, 28.

103 As a consequence the British patient is less likely: J. Mesker and P. Mesker, "Some Difficulties in Comparing Morbidity Between Countries," *Journal of the Royal College of General Practitioners* 29 (1979):92–96. M. von Cranach, "The Cross-National Comparability of Psychiatric Diagnoses," in *Cross-National Sociomedical Research: Concepts, Methods, Practice*, ed. Manfred Pflanz and Elisabeth Schach (Stuttgart: Georg Thieme, 1976); M. G. Sandifer, et al., "Similarities and Differences in Patient Evaluation by U.S. and U.K. Psychiatrists," *American Journal of Psychiatry* 126 (1969):206–12; Robin M. Murray, "A Reappraisal of American Psychiatry," *The Lancet*, Feb. 3, 1979, 255–58; "Editorial: Risks of Antihypertensive Therapy," *The Lancet*, Nov. 8, 1986, 1075–76. Canadian

recommendations for the treatment of high blood pressure are more similar to British practices, with the Canadian Hypertension Society now recommending drug therapy for diastolic blood pressure above 100 mm Hg., J. Cotter, "Use Drug Therapy on Diastolic BP Over 100 mm Hg," *The Medical Post*, June 26, 1984, 43.

104 The usual American interpretation: Aaron and Schwartz, *Painful Prescription*, provide a somewhat more sophisticated version of this interpretation, in that they recognize that the rationing is not uniform. But they don't emphasize those areas where the English expend more time and effort. For a critique of Aaron and Schwartz, see Frances H. Miller and Graham A. H. Miller, "The Painful Prescription: A Procrustean Perspective," *New England Journal of Medicine* 314 (1986):1383–86.

104 Certainly, there is . . . rationing: *Compendium of Health Statistics*, 4th ed. (London: Office of Health Economics, 1981), 22. The lengths of waiting lists are of course well known: "Brits Must Wait Up to 8 Months for Operations," *The Medical Post*, Mar. 19, 1985.

105 But not all the English economies: A. R. Henderson et al., "Letter: Clinical Chemistry Usage in Britain and Canada," *New England Journal of Medicine* 303 (1980):113–14; "British Oncologists Tepid on Adjuvants," *Oncology News*, Jan.–Feb. 1983; D. S. Greer, "Editorial," *Comparative Health Systems Newsletter* 8, no. 2 (Oct. 1986).

105 One explanation for British medical economy: "British Study Points Finger at 'Lazy GPs,' " *The Medical Post*, Feb. 19, 1985. A comparison of English and Canadian doctors found that while in England, 80 percent of general practitioners took vacations of five or six weeks, only one-third of Canadian general practitioners stayed away that long. J. Henahan, "English and Canadian MDs Aren't the Same," *The Medical Post*, July 27, 1982, 16.

106 Specialists are salaried: In 1984, about five million persons, or less than 10 percent of the population, were covered with private health insurance. "Why the Insurers Were the First to Put the Brakes on Costs," *The Times* (London), June 14, 1984, 17.

106 So in contrast to other countries: D. J. Hall, *The Relationship Between General Practitioners and Hospital Doctors, with Particular Reference to the Referral of Patients*, report to Department of Health and Social Security (London, 1979); B. Jennet, "How Many Specialists?" *The Lancet*, Mar. 17, 1979, 594–97; "Letter," *The Lancet*, Mar. 31, 1979, 729; N. Timmines, "GPs Prescribe an End to Patients' Sick Notes," *The Times* (London), June 19, 1981.

106 This system . . . was not suddenly imposed: For more information about the friendly societies, see Brian Abel-Smith, *The Hospitals in England and Wales, 1800–1948* (Cambridge, Mass.: Harvard University Press, 1964).

107 "Most British doctors . . .": B. Shurlock, "In England, the Royal Homeopath Helps Keep Unorthodox Medicine Respectable," *The Medical Post*, Mar. 5, 1985, 84.

107 The medical school training: Salvador de Madariaga, *Englishmen, Frenchmen and Spaniards* (New York: Hill and Wang, 1930). The Englishman John Hunter said many years ago, "Don't think: try," as quoted in J. R. Forbes, "Myth and Mumpsimus," *The Lancet*, Aug. 31, 1946. Disraeli is reported to have advised reading biography because it was life without the theory (*New York Daily News*, July 28, 1987, 8). That the English don't value thought as much as, for example, the French, may explain why English psychiatrists recognized thought disorders less often than the French and Germans in a three-way comparison. R. E. Kendell, Pierre Pichot, and M. von Cranach, "Diagnostic Criteria of English, French and German Psychiatrists," *Psychological Medicine* 4 (1974):187–95.

108 Thought derived of past experience: Henry Adams, *The Education of Henry Adams* (1907; reprint, New York: Modern Library, 1931), 453.

108 Dr. Maurice Mercadier: Maurice Mercadier, "Surgery, an International Discipline," *American Journal of Surgery* 150 (1985):237–38; Margaret Mead, "Some Problems of Cross-Cultural Communication between Britain and the United States: Based upon Lecturing in Britain and the United States during World War II," in *Study of Culture at a Distance*, ed. M. Mead and R. Métraux (Chicago: University of Chicago Press, 1953).

109 According to Dr. James V. O'Brien: James V. O'Brien, "It's into the Deep End in the UK," *The Medical Post*, Oct. 9, 1979.

109 This respect for factual details: J. L. Turk and Elizabeth Allen, "Bleeding and Cupping," *Annals of the Royal College of Surgeons of England*, 65 (1983):128–31.

110 The Victorian amateur scientist Francis Galton: Pierre Pichot, *A Century of Psychiatry* (Paris: Éditions Roger Dacosta, 1983); George Bernard Shaw, preface to *The Doctor's Dilemma* (1906; reprint, London: Penguin, 1977).

110 While clinical trials: In the Hypertension Detection and Follow-up Program study in the United States, for example, use of a placebo was considered unethical, and patients being treated by their family doctors were used as controls. In the British Medical Research Council study, placebos were used. Hypertension Detection and Follow-up Program Cooperative Group, "Five-year findings of the Hypertension Detection and Follow-up Program. I. Reduction in mortality of persons with high blood pressure, including mild hypertension," *Journal of the American Medical Association* 242 (1979):2562–71, and "Five-year findings of the Hypertension Detection and Follow-up Program. II. Mortality by race, sex and age," *Journal of the American Medical Association* 242 (1979):2572–77; Medical Research Council Working Party, "MRC trial of treatment of mild hypertension: principal results," *British Medical Journal* 291

(1985):97–104; J. Corrigan, "U.S. Hypertension Trial 'Absurdly Designed,' " *The Medical Post*, Oct. 19, 1982, 56.

110 The other difference is: Editorial, "Hypercholesterolaemia and Coronary Heart Disease: An Answer," *British Medical Journal* 288 (1984):423–24; Philip M. Boffey, "Study Backs Cutting Cholesterol to Curb Heart Disease," *The New York Times*, Jan. 13, 1984, 1; "Millions of Mild Hypertensives," *British Medical Journal* 281 (1980):1024; A. S. Relman, "Mild Hypertension: No More Benign Neglect," *New England Journal of Medicine* 302 (1980):293–94; A. Breckenridge, "Treating Mild Hypertension," *British Medical Journal* 291 (1985):89–90; S. Manek et al., "Persistence of Divergent Views of Hospital Staff in Detecting and Managing Hypertension," *British Medical Journal* 289 (1984):1433–34; "Hypertension in the Over-60s," *The Lancet*, June 28, 1980, 1396–97; "Transatlantic Contrasts: the BMA at San Diego," *British Medical Journal* 283 (1981):1234–39.

111 British doctors are also more likely: Earl Damude, "Study to Prove Effects of Amniocentesis," *The Medical Post*, Apr. 7, 1981; Helen Bantock and Ian Sutherland, "Risks of Amniocentesis," *British Medical Journal*, Oct. 13, 1979, 933–34; A. Colling et al., "Teesside Coronary Survey: An Epidemiologic Study of Acute Attacks of Myocardial Infarction," *British Medical Journal*, Nov. 13, 1976; M. H. Hall, P. K. Chng, and I. MacGillivray, "Is Routine Antenatal Care Worth While?" *The Lancet*, July 12, 1980, 78–80.

111 criticisms of periodic examinations: H. G. Turney, "Periodical Medical Examination," address to the Life Insurance Physicians of London, *The Lancet*, Feb. 18, 1928; G. C. Wilkinson and R. Pearson, "Letter: Well Man Clinic in General Practice," *British Medical Journal* 288 (1984):642–43.

112 English patients . . . tend to know little: C. M. Boyle, "Differences Between Patients' and Doctors' Interpretation of Some Common Medical Terms," *British Medical Journal*, May 2, 1970, 286–89.

112 In response to a more recent survey: Christianne Heal, "Letter: Anatomy Quiz," *Self Health* 3 (June 1984):34.

112 But another writer suggested: K. Spencer, "Letter: Anatomy Quiz," *Self Health* 3 (June 1984):34.

113 In a comparison with U.S. psychiatrists: The authors noted that it was usually a simple matter to distinguish between U.S. and U.K. reports from the raw data by merely noting the number of items checked. M. G. Sandifer et al., "Similarities and Differences in Patient Evaluation by U.S. and U.K. Psychiatrists," *American Journal of Psychiatry* 126 (1969):206–12. In the comparison of diagnostic criteria of English, French, and West German psychiatrists, agitation was rated far more often and thought disorder far less often by the English group than by French and German

psychiatrists. Some English psychiatrists also tended to rate weeping as a distinguishing feature of a depressive illness, and even of a manic-depressive illness. R. E. Kendell, P. Pichot, and M. von Cranach, "Diagnostic Criteria of English, French, and German Psychiatrists," *Psychological Medicine* 4 (1974):187–95. See also J. Leff, "International Variations in the Diagnosis of Psychiatric Illness," *International Journal of Psychiatry* 131 (1977):329–38; M. G. Sandifer et al., "Psychiatric Diagnosis: A Comparative Study in North Carolina, London and Glasgow," *British Journal of Psychiatry* 114 (1968):1–9; M. M. Katz, J. O. Cole, and H. A. Lowery, "Studies of the Diagnostic Process: The Influence of Symptoms Perception, Past Experience and Ethnic Background on Diagnostic Decisions," *American Journal of Psychiatry* 125 (1969):937–47.

British psychiatrists are much more likely to diagnose immigrants as schizophrenic than they are to give this label to native Britons. One study, for example, found that the diagnosis of schizophrenia was six times as common in Asian, African, and West Indian immigrants as in native Britons, although the diagnosis of neurotic depression was much more common among the native Britons. Immigrants of Eastern European origin, of which about half were Poles and Russians, had a rate of admission for schizophrenia four times higher than that for native Britons. One possible explanation, of course, is that delusions, considered one sign of schizophrenia, are extremely culture-bound. While an editorial in the *British Medical Journal* took the extreme differences in rates of schizophrenia diagnosis between Eastern Europeans and Britons to contradict the fact that the diagnosis of schizophrenia is being made incorrectly due to unfamiliarity with the cultural backgrounds—since "British psychiatrists might be expected only rarely to be mistaken and misidentify paranoid delusions in East European immigrants, since their respective cultural backgrounds are not dissimilar"—my thesis, of course, is that cultural backgrounds within Europe itself are not necessarily all that similar. "Paranoia and Immigrants," *British Medical Journal* 281 (1980): 1513–14. See also J. K. Wing, "International Comparisons in the Study of the Functional Psychoses," *British Medical Bulletin* 27, no. 1 (1971):77–81. In a comparison with Turkish patients, Turkish patients were found to have higher scores for delusions of grandeur, while English patients had higher ones for delusions of contrition. E. Gilleard, "A Cross-Cultural Investigation of Foulds' Hierarchy Model of Psychiatric Illness," *British Journal of Psychiatry* 142 (1983):518–23. Similarly, in another study, British patients were more intropunitive than Greek patients, and the Greek patients were more extrapunitive. G. C. Lyketsos, I. M. Blackburn, and D. Mouzaki, "Personality Variables and Dysthymic Symptoms: A Comparison Between a Greek and a British Sample," *Psychological Medicine* 9 (1979):753–58.

For an historical overview of English melancholia, see Vieda Skultans, *English Madness* (London, Boston, and Henley: Routledge & Kegan Paul, 1979).

113 Tranquillizer use . . . relatively high: M. B. Balter, J. Levine, and D. I. Manheimer, "Cross-National Study of the Extent of Anti-Anxiety/Sedative Drug Use," *New England Journal of Medicine* 290 (1974):769–74; O'Brien, *Patterns of European Diagnoses*; "Editorial: Beta-Blockers in Situational Anxiety," *The Lancet*, July 27, 1985, 193.

113 Over 2 percent: O'Brien, *Patterns of European Diagnoses*; P. Tyrer, "Drug Treatment of Psychiatric Patients in General Practice," *British Medical Journal*, Oct. 7, 1978, 1008–10.

114 Several English doctors: R. Birenbaum, "Psychotropic Prescriptions a GP Timesaver?" *The Journal*, Jan. 1, 1981; Cecil G. Helman, "Patients' Perceptions of Psychotropic Drugs," *Journal of the Royal College of General Practitioners* 31 (1981):107–12.

115 A similar concern about self-control: C. Brewer, "Letter: Royal Organs," *British Medical Journal*, Mar. 15, 1980, 794; *Compendium of Health Statistics*, 4th ed. (London: Office of Health Economics, 1981), 22. In 1982, about 155 kilograms of heroin were used in Great Britain, mostly for the treatment of pain, compared to 57 kilograms in 1975. Testimony given by H. B. Spear, chief inspector of the Home Office in Great Britain, in hearings of the House subcommittee on health, Mar. 8, 1984, chaired by Henry Waxman. I suspect that the stiff-upper-lip mentality may explain the relatively greater enthusiasm shown by British doctors for both electroconvulsive therapy and psychosurgery. While the British general practitioner who treated one in seven of his patients with ECT, including those with rheumatoid arthritis, was forced to quit (H. Griffiths, " 'Shock' Doctor Forced to Quit," *The Medical Post*, Nov. 27, 1984), ECT remains fairly acceptable to British psychiatrists. While electroconvulsive therapy has all but disappeared from many countries, British psychiatrists remain enthusiastic, calling the evidence that the treatment is effective for severe depressive illness "substantial and incontrovertible" (R. E. Kendall, "Electroconvulsive Therapy," *Journal of the Royal Society of Medicine* 71 [1978]: 319–21). For a discussion of the use of neurosurgery for psychological disorder, see B. M. Barraclough and N. A. Mitchell-Heggs, "Use of Neurosurgery for Psychological Disorder in British Isles during 1974–76," *British Medical Journal* 2 (Dec. 9, 1978):1591–93. A 1984 study found that over 75 percent of psychiatrists working in two areas requested psychosurgical facilities for the referral of patients. R. P. Snaith, D. J. E. Price, and J. F. Wright, "Psychiatrists' Attitudes to Psychosurgery: Proposals for the Organization of a Psychosurgical Service in Yorkshire," *British Journal of Psychiatry* 144 (1984):293–97.

116 "From infancy . . .": "Editorial: Investigating Constipation," *British Medical Journal*, Mar. 8, 1980, 669–70; Jonathan Miller, *The Body in Question* (New York: Random House, 1978); "World Health Organization International Collaborative Study of Medical Care Utilization," ed. Robert

Kohn and Kerr White (London, New York: Oxford University Press, 1976).

116 When an Englishman talks about his liver: Boyle, "Interpretation of Medical Terms."

116 Constipation perhaps really is . . . a problem: Liselotte Hojgaard et al., "Tea Consumption: A Cause of Constipation?" *British Medical Journal* 282 (1981):864.

116 But the English may also perceive more constipation: Boyle, "Interpretation of Medical Terms."

117 At least part of this obsession: Edward C. Lambert, *Modern Medical Mistakes* (Bloomington: Indiana University Press, 1978); G. Dussault and A. Sheiham, "Medical Theories and Professional Development: The Theory of Focal Sepsis and Dentistry in Early Twentieth Century Britain," *Social Science and Medicine* 16 (1982):1405–12; Shaw, *Doctor's Dilemma*.

117 While the theory of autointoxication: Denis P. Burkitt, "Etiology and Prevention of Colorectal Cancer," *Hospital Practice*, Feb. 1984, 67–77; "Editorial: Investigating Constipation," *British Medical Journal*, Mar. 8, 1980, 669–70; "Minerva," "Views," *British Medical Journal*, Jan. 7, 1978, 54.

117 The answer to my question: Michael O'Donnell, "The Health Trait that Marks an Englishman," *The Medical Post*, Feb. 18, 1986, 36. According to film critic John Lownsbrough, reviewing the movie *A Private Function*, while American humor has tended to fix on sex, English humor has seemed to derive a special delight from matters relating to the toilet. John Lownsbrough, "Status the Thing in This Class Act," *The Medical Post*, Apr. 30, 1985, 30.

118 Compared to the French and Germans: O'Brien, *Patterns of European Diagnoses*; A. M. W. Porter and J. M. T. Porter, "Anglo-French Contrasts in Medical Practice," *British Medical Journal*, Apr. 26, 1980, 1109–12.

118 Unlike French women: Rory Williams, "Concepts of Health: An Analysis of Lay Logic," *Sociology* 17 (1983):185–205.

118 This sort of corporeal xenophobia: Luigi Barzini, *The Europeans* (New York: Simon and Schuster, 1983); J. Wetz, "On ne badine pas avec la rage," *Le Monde*, July 25–26, 1976, 11; D. Fitzpatrick, "The Light at the End of the Chunnel?" *MD*, Sept. 1986, 55–58; "Minerva," "Views," *British Medical Journal* 290 (1985):1830; D. Armstrong, et al., "Letter: British AIDS Regulations Show an Uninformed Response," *The New York Times*, Apr. 4, 1985; J. F. Clarity, "Britain Begins Crash Campaign to Educate Public About the Spread of AIDS," *The New York Times*, Jan. 29, 1987, B24; "Knowledge Lessens AIDS Fears," *The Medical Post*, Sept.

23, 1986, 24; "Firemen Told: Don't 'Kiss' Homosexuals," *The Medical Post,* Apr. 2, 1985, 1.

119 One favorite environmental explanation: A. S. Robertson et al., "Comparison of Health Problems Related to Work and Environmental Measurements in Two Office Buildings with Different Ventilation Systems," *British Medical Journal* 291 (1985):373–76; C. G. Helman, " 'Feed a Cold, Starve a Fever'—Folk Models of Infection in an English Suburban Community, and their Relation to Medical Treatment," *Culture, Medicine and Psychiatry* 2 (1978):107–37; C. G. Helman, "General Practitioner as Social Anthropologist," *British Medical Journal* 282 (1981):787–88.

119 Chills, of course, may lead to chilblains: B. E. Beacham et al., "Equestrian Cold Panniculitis in Women," *Archives of Dermatology* 116 (1980):1025–27; Renwick Vickers, "Letter: Equestrian Cold Panniculitis," *British Medical Journal* 282 (1981):405.

120 In fact, while the British: Derek Robinson, "Primary Medical Practice in the United Kingdom and the United States," *New England Journal of Medicine* 297 (1977):188–93; K. McRae, "Geriatrics a Growing Specialty in UK," *The Medical Post,* Aug. 1, 1978; Thomas Pickering, "The Future of Cardiology and Psychogeriatrics," *British Medical Journal* 283 (1981):377, and responses, ibid., 494–96, 671–72, 791.

121 Kindness can also be seen: T. B. Brewin, "Uncritical Appraisal of Cancer Chemotherapy," *British Medical Journal* 290 (1985):232–33; Jean McCann, "Briton Resists American Adjuvant Cancer Dogma," *The Medical Post,* May 1, 1984. Hormonal therapy (with many fewer side effects) for breast cancer was popular in Britain at a time when chemotherapy was still the dogma in the United States; and it was later proven to be just as effective as the chemotherapy. Many would say that the fact that arthritics in Britain are more likely to be treated with nonsteroidal anti-inflammatory drugs other than aspirin is due to the fact that these newer drugs have fewer side effects than aspirin.

121 The lesser belief in medicine's ability: F. M. Hull, "Quality and Quantity in Primary Medical Care," *Update,* June 1976, 1287–91.

121 "There is a fit . . .": D. H. Smith and J. A. Granbois, "The American Way of Hospice," *Hastings Center Report,* Apr. 1982, 8–10.

122 But the caring is often paternalistic: Harvey McConnell, "British Get Protection from 'Informed Consent,' " *The Medical Post,* Apr. 3, 1984; Robert Schwartz and Andrew Grubb, "Why Britain Can't Afford Informed Consent," *Hastings Center Report,* Aug. 1985, 19–25; P. S. Appelbaum, "England's New Commitment Law," *Hospital and Community Psychiatry* 36 (1985):705–13.

122 One study found: "British Patients Fear They'll Annoy MDs," *The Medical Post,* Aug. 24, 1982.

United States

Page

124 "In short . . .": Logan Clendening, *The Care and Feeding of Adults* (New York: Alfred A. Knopf, 1931).

124 Prophylactic removal of both breasts: J. W. Alderson, "An Indecent Proposal," *Mother Jones*, May 1985, 52–56; Ann Todd, "Prophylactic Mastectomy," *American Journal of Nursing*, Sept. 1977, 1447–49.

124 American medicine is aggressive: C. Francome and P. J. Huntingford, "Births by Caesarean Section in the United States of America and in Britain," *Journal of Biosocial Science* 12 (1980): 353–62; F. C. Notzon, P. J. Placek, and S. M. Taffel, "Comparisons of National Cesarean-Section Rates," *New England Journal of Medicine* 316 (1987):386–89; "C-Sections Continue to Increase in U.S." *New York Daily News*, Jan. 26, 1987, 7 extra. S. B. Thacker and H. D. Banta, "Benefits and Risks of Episiotomy: An Interpretative Review of the English Language Literature, 1860–1980," *Obstetrical and Gynecological Survey* 38 (1983):322–38; W. A. Knaus et al., "A Comparison of Intensive Care in the U.S.A. and in France," *The Lancet*, Sept. 18, 1982, 642–46; S. A. Schroeder, "A Comparison of Western European and U.S. University Hospitals: A Case Report from Leuven, West Berlin, Leiden, London and San Francisco," *Journal of the American Medical Association*, 252 (1984):240–46; for surgery rates in general, see note to page 24; P. J. DiSaia and W. T. Creasman, *Clinical Gynecologic Oncology* (St. Louis, Toronto, Princeton: C. V. Mosby, 1984). Despite the publicity given to less mutilating treatments for breast cancer, in the early 1980s most women were still being treated with a modified version of the radical mastectomy, *Health United States* (Washington, D.C.: U.S. Government Printing Office, 1985), Samuel Shem, *The House of God* (New York: Dell, 1979).

125 American doctors perform more diagnostic tests: G. N. Marsh, R. B. Wallace, and J. Whewell, "Anglo-American Contrasts in General Practice," *British Medical Journal*, May 29, 1976, 1321–25; Eleanor Moskovic, "Massachusetts General Hospital," *British Medical Journal* 283 (1981):1242–44. The standard dose for Rh immune globulin in North America is 300 micrograms, whereas in other parts of the world it is 100 to 125 micrograms. J. M. Bowman, "Controversies in Rh Prophylaxis," *American Journal of Obstetrics and Gynecology* 151 (1985):289–94; Olga Lechky, "Many MDs Exceeding Anticoagulant Guidelines," *The Medical Post*, Nov. 12, 1985, 26; R. Faizallah et al., "Is There a Place in the United Kingdom for Intensive Antacid Treatment for Chronic Peptic Ulceration?" *British Medical Journal* 289 (1984):869–71; "Hyperkinetic Kids Getting 4 Times Too Many Stimulants," *The Medical Post*, Apr. 10, 1979.

125 The dosages in psychiatry are particularly high: H.-U. Fisch, J. S. Gillis, and R. Daguet, "A Cross-National Study of Drug Treatment Decisions

in Psychiatry," *Medical Decision Making* 2 (1982):167–77; Dava Sobel, "Something Nasty at the Bottom of the Psychiatric Drug Bottle," *The New York Times*, June 8, 1980.

125 Surgery . . . besides being performed more often: Centers for Disease Control, "Surgical Sterilization Surveillance: Hysterectomy in Women Aged 15–44, 1976–78," Mar. 1981; E. Vayda, W. R. Mindell, and L. M. Rutkow, "A Decade of Surgery in Canada, England and Wales, and the United States," *Archives of Surgery* 117 (1982):846–53. E. R. Novak, G. S. Jones, and H. W. Jones, Jr., *Novak's Textbook of Gynecology*, 9th ed. (Baltimore: Williams and Wilkins, 1975); Göran Larsson, "The Conization Operation and Its Predecessors," *Acta Obstetrica Gynecologica Scandinavica Supplementa* 114 (1983):7–40. While the 1981 edition of *Novak's Textbook of Gynecology* no longer supported hysterectomy across the board for all women, admitting that "hysterectomy is an operation which, in some quarters, has acquired an onerous reputation, due perhaps to a small minority of overzealous surgeons (frequently not gynecologists) who have seemed inclined to believe that removal of the uterus would be the panacea for every pain or discomfort which might afflict the woman. A constructive but critical report by D'Espopo would indicate that most hysterectomies performed by specialists are *justifiable even though the uterus shows no evidence of a pathological condition*" (italics mine). The book also said that if hysterectomy was performed, "our inclination is toward the radical approach, namely removal of the gonads if the patient is over about 40 years of age."

126 Prostate surgery also: R. J. C. Pearson et al., "Hospital Caseloads in Liverpool, New England and Uppsala"; "The Case Against Neonatal Circumcision," *British Medical Journal*, May 5, 1979, 1163–64; J. L. Wirth, "Statistics on Circumcision in Canada and Australia," *American Journal of Obstetrics and Gynecology* 130 (1978):236–39.

126 Public health policies on vaccination: For a comparison and critique of the different rubella strategies, see *The Lancet*, June 23, 1979, 1329–31.

126 Many conditions, such as high blood pressure: G. E. Thomson et al., "High Blood Pressure Diagnosis and Treatment: Consensus Recommendations vs. Actual Practice," *American Journal of Public Health* 71 (1981):413–16; Hypertension Detection and Follow-up Program Cooperative Group, "Five-year Findings of the Hypertension Detection and Follow-up Program. Reduction in Mortality of Persons with High Blood Pressure, Including Mild Hypertension," *Journal of American Medical Association* 242 (1979):2562–71; Jean McCann, "New Guidelines May Mean Half U.S. Has High BP," *The Medical Post*, Oct. 19, 1982, 33.

126 Even when American medicine leans: "Hyperlipidemia Should Be Aggressively Treated," *The Medical Post*, June 12, 1984, 22. Dr. Howard Morgan, president of the American Heart Association, used the words "aggressive" or "aggressively" five times in an address to the American

Heart Association's Delegate Assembly on June 21, 1987, in Dallas, Texas. After a mentally retarded man died at a New York State hospital after doctors tried, without consent, to amputate his healthy legs to obtain skin grafts to repair bedsores on his body, a hospital spokeswoman was quoted as saying that the hospital was "actually proud of the aggressive measures we took to save his life." K. Kerr, *New York Daily News*, June 9, 1987, 6; P. M. Boffey, "U.S. Seeks to Curb Reliance on Drugs for Blood Pressure," *The New York Times*, May 1, 1984, A1.

126 when a twelve-hospital study . . . found: Eric Eckholm, "Gentle Method Proves Better for Premature Babies' Lungs," *The New York Times*, Jan. 6, 1987, C3.

127 This medical aggressiveness: Oliver Wendell Holmes, *Medical Essays, 1842–1882* (Boston: Houghton Mifflin, 1888); R. C. Toth, "What Makes Americans Different? Study Lists 10 Significant—and Lasting—Traits," *International Herald Tribune*, Oct. 3, 1977, 9.

127 The aggressive approach that has characterized: John Duffy, *The Healers: A History of American Medicine* (New York: McGraw-Hill, 1976). Quote about Rush feeling that nature had been put under control of the American revolution came from Oliver Wendell Holmes, via N. E. Davies, G. H. Davies, and E. D. Sanders, "William Cobbett, Benjamin Rush and the Death of General Washington," *Journal of the American Medical Association* 249 (1983):912–15.

128 Another historian, Martin S. Pernick: M. S. Pernick, "The Calculus of Suffering in Nineteenth-Century Surgery," *Hastings Center Report*, Apr. 1983, 26–36.

129 When France became the mecca of medical progress: John Harley Warner, "The Selective Transport of Medical Knowledge: Antebellum American Physicians and Parisian Medical Therapeutics," *Bulletin of the History of Medicine* 59 (1985):213–31; see also E. H. Ackerknecht, *A Short History of Medicine* (Baltimore: Johns Hopkins University Press, 1982), 221–22.

129 The tendency to favor aggressive therapy: Margarete Sandelowski, *Pain, Pleasure, and American Childbirth: From the Twilight Sleep to the Read Method, 1914–1960* (Westport, Conn.: Greenwood Press, 1984).

130 Cesarean section is now: R. C. Wright, "Editorial: Hysterectomy: Past, Present and Future," *Obstetrics and Gynecology* 35 (1969):560–63. Novak et al., *Novak's Textbook*. The tendency is not limited to male gynecologists: in her address to the thirty-third annual meeting of the South Atlantic Association of Obstetricians and Gynecologists, Eleanor B. Easley outlined many typically American reasons for hysterectomy: "In many ways hysterectomy fits women's present needs. It is an excellent procedure for sterilization. A woman is a more reliable worker after she's had one.

It is advantageous at the menopause if only to simplify estrogen therapy. For some time I've been telling women that in another twenty years I expect hysterectomy to have become almost routine at the menopause." Eleanor B. Easley, "The Dilemma of Women in Our Culture: Gynecologic Repercussions: Part II," *American Journal of Obstetrics and Gynecology* 110 (1971):858–64.

Further evidence that Americans believe nature is something to conquer: Unlike regulations in Britain, West Germany, and Scandinavia, rules governing pilot scheduling in the United States don't take circadian rhythms into account. According to Dr. Joseph G. Constantino, the chairman of the International Air Transport Association and corporate medical director for Pan American, "Pilots are professional travelers and have learned how to cope with jet lag by setting their own body clocks." Nancy J. Perry, "Industrial Time Clocks—Often at Odds with Those Inside a Worker's Body," *The New York Times*, Nov. 28, 1982, F8–F9. A similar situation prevails with regard to studies showing that certain drugs should be given at certain times of day. Lisa Davis, "Timing Is Everything," *Hippocrates* July/Aug. 1987, 22.

131 "Pragmatic Americans...": Luigi Barzini, *The Europeans* (New York: Simon and Schuster, 1983).

131 All this trying to do something: M. Searle, "Obsessive-Compulsive Behaviour in American Medicine," *Social Science and Medicine* 15E (1981):185–93; Moskovic, "Massachusetts General Hospital"; B. S. Sandhu, "Personal View," *British Medical Journal* 285 (1982):287.

132 But all this rushing about: Charcot quoted in Pierre Pichot, *A Century of Psychiatry* (Paris: Editions Roger Dacosta, 1983). In a 1984 report from Philip Hendrix at Emory University, 40 percent of the U.S. population was classed as "harried."

132 Another victim: Ronald Gelfand and Frank Kline, "Differences in Diagnostic Patterns in Britain and America," *Comprehensive Psychiatry* 19 (1978):551–55. Medicare was intended only to insure against illnesses that were being actively treated. L. Saxe, "The Effectiveness and Costs of Alcoholism Treatment," Washington, D.C.: Office of Technology Assessment, Health Technology Case Study 22.

133 "When you refer": W. Abberman, "Letter: Victors Over Cancer," *The New York Times Magazine*, Mar. 11, 1984, 142.

133 Those who refuse treatment: G. J. Annas, "Prisoner in the ICU: The Tragedy of William Bartling," *Hastings Center Report*, Dec. 1984, 28–29.

133 Dr. Klass, writing of her Harvard Medical School education: Perri Klass, "Bearing a Child in Medical School," *The New York Times Magazine*, Nov. 11, 1984.

134 The same clinical trials: Hypertension Detection and Follow-up Program Cooperative Group, "Five-year Findings . . . Reduction of Mortality"; T. G. Pickering, "Treatment of Mild Hypertension and the Reduction of Cardiovascular Mortality: The 'of or by' dilemma," *Journal of the American Medical Association* 249 (1983):399–400.

134 When pressed . . . American doctors often answer: Malpractice, of course, is one mechanism by which the culture values determine medical treatment. That American juries may be kinder on the doctor whose sins were of commission, rather than of omission, has some support; see, for example, H. Eisenberg, "A Doctor on Trial," *New York Times Magazine*, July 20, 1986, 26–42, where a jury found an obstetrician guilty because during a difficult delivery he hadn't broken the baby's collar bone, which might have eased the delivery. But malpractice is not by any means the only reason American doctors are aggressive. One study found that while the threat of malpractice made many doctors order more diagnostic tests, it was less likely to make them limit the procedures they undertook: they interpreted the threat of malpractice as being not doing enough rather than doing things they perhaps weren't qualified to do. Ferris J. Ritchey, "Medical Rationalization, Cultural Lag and the Malpractice Crisis," *Human Organization* 40 (1981):97–111. Countries such as Germany and Australia, which have similarly aggressive national characters, fee-for-service medicine, *but* lower malpractice rates, nevertheless show high rates of procedures that are probably unnecessary. See Lois Quam, Robert Dingwall, and Paul Fenn, "Medical Malpractice in Perspective: The American Experience," *British Medical Journal* 294 (1987):1529–32, and Eric E. Fortess and Marshall B. Kapp, "Medical Uncertainty, Diagnostic Testing, and Legal Liability," *Law, Medicine and Health Care* 13 (1985):213–18.

134 The threat of malpractice: Philip R. Liebson and Michael H. Davidson, "Mitral Valve Prolapse: Recent Advances in Diagnosis and Therapy," *Comprehensive Therapy*, June 1987, 21–32.

135 In one university hospital: K. Steel et al., "Iatrogenic Illness on a General Medical Service at a University Hospital," *New England Journal of Medicine* 304 (1981):638–42; J. R. A. Mitchell, "First We Debilitate, Then We Rehabilitate," *British Medical Journal*, Nov. 3, 1979, 1132–33. A study at the University of Miami School of Medicine found that about one-third of ischemic strokes occurring in the hospital could be classed as iatrogenic, with overly aggressive acute management of hypertension the major offender. A. Rand, "Strokes Linked to BP 'Cure,' " *The Medical Post*, June 28, 1983, 1. A doctor "slowdown" in Los Angeles County, California, that consisted mostly in withholding elective surgery was accompanied by a decline in the death rate—followed by a sharp rise when surgery was resumed. M. I. Roemer, "More Data on Post-Surgical Deaths Related to the 1976 Los Angeles Doctor Slowdown," *Social Science and Medicine* 15C (1981):161–63. Certain deaths and brain damage have been linked to the practice of using routine intravenous therapy after

surgery, leading to low salt levels in the body. Sandra Blakeslee, "Low Salt Levels Linked to Death," *The New York Times*, June 12, 1986. A paper by D. H. Lawson and H. Jick that compared patients in the United States and Scotland found that Scottish patients on the average received half the drugs in hospital that U.S. patients did. Twenty-eight percent of the American patients had one or more adverse effects attributed to drug treatment, as compared to 21 percent of Scots. Two California scientists estimated in 1974 that from 60,000 to 140,000 deaths occur annually in U.S. hospitals due to adverse reactions to drugs. Morton Mintz, "U.S. Experts Boost Estimate on Drug Deaths in Hospitals," *The Washington Post*, May 21, 1974.

136 A group led by Nathan Couch: N. P. Couch et al., "The High Cost of Low-Frequency Events," *New England Journal of Medicine* 304 (1981):634–37.

136 And while the can-do approach: P. M. Boffey, "Cancer Survival Rate Progress Is Reported, But Skeptics Object," *The New York Times*, Nov. 27, 1984, C1. "NIH Questioned over Cancer Research," *IMS Pharmaceutical Marketletter*, June 19, 1978, 3. A. Geddes, "Measles May Be Unbeatable, Congress Is Told," *The Medical Post*, Oct. 16, 1984; J. C. Jacobs, "Letters: Much Ado About Pupils' Immunization," *The New York Times*, Oct. 17, 1981, 154; P. J. Imperato, "Letters: The High Cost of Attempting to Rid America of Measles," *The New York Times*, Oct. 28, 1981, 152.

137 Defeats never seem to call into doubt: Annette Oestreicher, "ACOG Backs Fetal Monitoring Despite Tie to More Cesareans," *Medical Tribune*, June 18, 1980, 3; Edward Edelson, "Breast Cancer Study Disputes Diet Theory," *New York Daily News*, Jan. 5, 1987, 12 extra; Edward Edelson, "Cancer Experts Chew the Fat—and Call for Lots Less," *New York Daily News*, Mar. 26, 1987, 38.

137 As a consequence . . . Americans are not: P. J. Strauss, "Letter: Alzheimer's Is Bankrupting U.S. Families," *The New York Times*, Sept. 19, 1985; J. Haas, "Rehabilitation: No Organ to Stand On," *Hastings Center Report*, Aug. 1986, 46–47; S. Kaufman and G. Becker, "Stroke: Health Care on the Periphery," *Social Science and Medicine* 22 (1986):983–89; "Studies Show U.S. Arthritis Sufferers Not Receiving Good Care," *The Medical Post*, Sept. 14, 1976, 24; Robin Herman, "Geriatric Psychiatry Is Much Enfeebled," *The New York Times*, Jan. 27, 1980.

138 The penchant for doing things fast: "Synovectomy for Rheumatoid Arthritis: Pretesting New Substances for Toxicity," *Journal of the American Medical Association* 240 (1978):2041.

139 Similarly, studies of what works: Richard Lyons, "How Release of Mental Patients Began," *The New York Times*, Oct. 30, 1984, C1; W. T. Carpenter, T. H. McGlashan, and J. S. Strauss, "The Treatment of Acute Schizophrenia Without Drugs: An Investigation of Some Current Assumptions," *American Journal of Psychiatry* 134 (1977):14–20; J. Brinkley,

"More Risk in Surgery of Prostate," *The New York Times*, Jan. 6, 1987, A14.

139 Probably as a result, Americans have . . . a passion for diagnosis: Shem, *House of God*.

139 Alistair Cooke notes: Alistair Cooke, "The Doctor in Society," *British Medical Journal* 283 (1981):19–26; H. M. Cameron, Euphemia Mc-Googan, and Helen Watson, "Necropsy: A Yardstick for Clinical Diagnoses," *British Medical Journal* 281 (1980):985–88; Tobias Kircher, Judith Nelson, and Harold Burdo, "The Autopsy as a Measure of Accuracy of the Death Certificate," *New England Journal of Medicine* 313 (1985):1263–69.

140 The search for a diagnosis: Stanley J. Reiser, *Medicine and the Reign of Technology* (New York: Cambridge University Press, 1978).

140 A patient seeing a GP: Marsh et al., "Anglo-American Contrasts in General Practice," *British Medical Journal*, May 29, 1976, 1321–25; L. S. Linn et al., "Differences in the Numbers and Costs of Tests Ordered by Internists, Physicians and Psychiatrists," *Inquiry* 21 (Fall 1984):266–75.

140 In hospital, too: George E. Lindhardt, Jr., Robert Moore, and J. Laurence Hill, "Comparison of Health Care Delivery in Britain and the United States," *Maryland State Medical Journal*, July 1982, 41–45; Schroeder, "Comparison of Hospitals"; W. A. Knaus et al., "A Comparison of Intensive Care in the U.S.A. and in France," *The Lancet*, Sept. 18, 1982, 642–46.

141 Eleanor Moskovic: Moskovic, "Massachusetts General Hospital."

141 Many Americans, of course: "More Physician Probing, Fewer Lab Tests for Diagnoses Urged," *The Medical Post*, Feb. 27, 1979, 7.

141 "I am convinced . . .": Mike Oppenheim, "Healers," *New England Journal of Medicine* 303 (1980):1117–20.

142 Not only is such testing expensive: "Comment: Foetal Biophysic Monitoring: Its Effects on the Cesarean Section and Perinatal Mortality Frequency," *Obstetrical and Gynecological Survey* 37 (Mar. 1982): 179–80.

142 Similarly, the frequent screening: While my own gynecologist recommends the test yearly, the laboratory he uses sends out little cards that state, "It has been *at least* six months," implying that failure to act immediately will have dire consequences; Larsson, "The Conization Operation and Its Predecessors."

142 A California physician explained: Thomas Hill, "Pap Smear Controversy Splits World Congress," *The Medical Post*, Jan. 16, 1979, 21.

143 If, in spite of all the tests: E. G. Anderson, "The Perpetual Patient," *Physician East*, Oct. 1980, 19.

143 Alistair Cooke: Cooke, "Doctor in Society"; Sandra Blakeslee, "Folklore Mirrors Life's Key Themes," *The New York Times*, Aug. 14, 1985.

144 So strong is the belief: M. S. Keller, "Letters: Rx: Garlic and Onion," *Fortune*, Apr. 5, 1982, 22; May 3, 1982, 40.

144 While West German doctors would maintain: D. Cassels, "Population up 11 percent—Antibiotic Use Up 300 Percent," *The Medical Post*, June 6, 1978, 1. In one study of specialists in a community hospital, only 60 percent of antibiotic prescriptions were considered appropriate. G. J. Jogerst and S. E. Dippe, "Antibiotic Use Among Medical Specialties in a Community Hospital," *Journal of the American Medical Association* 245 (1981):842–46. D. H. Lawson and H. Jick, paper presented at the Seventh International Congress of Pharmacology, Paris, 1978; Bernie O'Brien, *Patterns of European Diagnoses and Prescribing* (London: Office of Health Economies, 1984); Jean McCann, "Antibiotic Overload May Spell Doom for Medical Use," *The Medical Post*, Aug. 1, 1978, 16.

144 The idea that disease must be caused: L. L. Wisdo, "Je Suis Americaine— Especially in Paris," *Columbia Magazine*, Nov. 1983, 21–26.

145 In an advertisement: "8 Ways to Strengthen Your Immune System," *Healthline*, Apr. 1984, 20–21; R. Trubo, "Toilet Terrors: What You Can/ Can't Catch in Bathrooms," *Self*, Sept. 1983, 122.

145 The American penchant for cleanliness: P. de Vries, "Patients Bring on ENT Complaints with Commercial Home Remedies," *The Medical Post*, Jan. 20, 1976, 8; "Intermenstrual Tampon Use Linked to Vaginal Ulcers," *The Medical Post*, May 19, 1981, 45; Novak et al., *Novak's Textbook*; Robert B. McLaren, "Circumcision: The Most Unneeded Surgery of All," *Medical Month*, Dec. 1983, 50–54; Cynthia Rand, Carol-Ann Emmons, and J. W. C. Johnson, "The Effect of an Educational Intervention on the Rate of Neonatal Circumcision," *Obstetrics and Gynecology* 62 (1983):64–68.

146 Dr. Robert E. Hodges: Robert Hodges, *Nutrition in Medical Practice* (Philadelphia: W. B. Saunders, 1980); "Iron Deficiency Laid to Fewer Iron Pots, Pans," *International Herald Tribune*, Aug. 31, 1973, 3.

146 Once a substance is branded: "Pregnant Women Shouldn't Drink at All: Panel," *The Journal*, Dec. 1, 1977; Edward Edelson, "2 Drinks No Pregnancy Risk?" *New York Daily News*, Oct. 4, 1983; K. Jenkins, "Four Drinks Will Not Harm Unborn Baby," *The Medical Post*, May 12, 1987, 1; Harvey McConnell, "Effects of Alcohol on Fetus Exaggerated," *The Medical Post*, Jan. 21, 1986.

147 Salt, which causes: Robert F. Capon, "In Praise of Salt, a Friend Maligned," *The New York Times*, Sept. 8, 1982, 6C; *Consumer Product Safety Network Newsletter* 2, no. 2 (May/June 1984); S. Roy III, "Perspectives on Adverse Effects of Milks and Infant Formulas Used in Infant Feeding," *Journal of the American Dietetic Association*, 82 (1983):373–77.

148   The preference for taking something out: John Kelly, "Bridging America's Drug Gap," *The New York Times Magazine*, Sept. 13, 1981, 100ff; information from the U.S. General Accounting Office (1975) quoted by the Upjohn Company.

148   That peculiarly American institution, the checkup: Reiser, *Medicine and the Reign of Technology*.

148   Body as car: M. Poriss, *How to Live Cheap But Good* (New York: Dell, 1971); H. Bloom, review of *In the Freud Archives* by Janet Malcolm, *The New York Times Book Review*, May 27, 1984, 3ff.; Janet Malcolm, *Psychoanalysis: The Impossible Profession* (New York: Knopf, 1981).

148   And in a recent letter: L. Schwarzbaum, "Letter: Maintaining the Body," *The New York Times Magazine*, Feb. 19, 1984, 94.

149   Perhaps it was an extreme application: R. B. Punkett, Jr., "Sex Organs, Breasts, Called Non $$ Productive," *New York Daily News*, Dec. 18, 1985.

149   The popularity of the idea of body as machine: T. A. Preston, *Coronary Artery Surgery: A Critical Review* (New York: Raven Press, 1977); J. Schaefer, "The Case Against Coronary Artery Surgery: A Paradigm for Studying the Nature of a So-called Scientific Controversy in the Field of Cardiology," *Metamedicine* 1 (1980):155–76; Dr. Thomas J. Ryan was quoted as saying, "I think the Holy Grail is the formulation of a medicine that one can take in pill form that will act as a cardiovascular Drano and clean out the pipes," in "Heart Disease Deaths Are Dropping, But Why?" *The New York Times*, Nov. 18, 1984.

149   When the operation was eventually studied: "Live Longer, Maybe; Live Better, Yes," *The Medical Post*, Dec. 13, 1983, 18; G. B. Kolata, "Consensus on Bypass Surgery," *Science*, 211 (1981):42–43.

150   A member of a panel who evaluated the operation: Kolata, "Consensus on Bypass Surgery."

150   In theory, the large proportion of psychiatrists: Robin M. Murray, "A Reappraisal of American Psychiatry," *The Lancet*, Feb. 3, 1979, 255–58. Michael O'Donnell, "It's the American Dream That's in Need of a Facelift," *The Medical Post*, Mar. 23, 1982, 24.

150   And in another . . . : Janet Malcolm, *In the Freud Archives* (New York: Knopf, 1984).

150   This approach . . . was probably inevitable: T. M. Johnson, "Medical Education and Practice on the Periphery: Consultation Psychiatry and the Psychosocial Tradition in American Medicine," *Social Science and Medicine* 22 (1986):963–71.

151   Bruno Bettelheim in his book: Bruno Bettelheim, *Freud and Man's Soul* (New York: Knopf, 1982).

151   This denial of the soul: Andree Brooks, "Childbearing Centers Are Increasing in Popularity," *The New York Times*, June 18, 1983.

152   When reporters asked of the artificial heart: D. Nelkin, *Selling Science* (New York: W. H. Freeman, 1987), 44.

152   The artificial hearts failed: P. J. Rosch, "Letter: Can an Artificial Heart Have Its Reasons?" *The New York Times*, Jan. 7, 1985.

Acknowledgments

Ten years ago I decided to write a book on the relatively un-focused subject of differences in medical treatment among de-veloped countries, and my agent from the outset, Eleanor Wood, deserves the most heartfelt thanks for suffering with me each time the vague idea took a new shape. I would also like to thank Peter Weed for recognizing early on that the idea could become a book, and to my editor Channa Taub for helping me finally make it one.

Along the way a number of people helped shape my thoughts, and I owe particular debts to Drs. Kerr White, Zoltan Zarday, Marcel-Francis Kahn, John P. Bunker, Thomas Pickering, Cecil Helman, Jean-Pierre Benhamou, Herbert Viefhues, F. M. Hull, Graham Dukes, Per Knut Lunde, and the late Manfred Pflanz. Many of these also critiqued the manuscript at various stages, and I would like to thank Drs. Peter Robra, Mack Lipkin, Jr., Jean-Pierre Armand, and Ilse King also for their critiques. In addition, I would like to thank all the doctors who graciously consented to be interviewed, particularly Dr. David Winstanley, who put me in contact with other members of the Anglo-German Medical Society. I am of course fully responsible for the accuracy of the information I cite.

Among the nondoctors who read the manuscript I would like to thank Gerald Geison, Ph.D., of the department of the history of science at Princeton University and Shelley Frisch, Ph.D., of the German department of Columbia University and several instructors at Deutsches Haus in New York. Thanks also to a number of my friends who read the manuscript, especially to Tom Reed, Nancy Festinger, Bertram Schwarzschild, and Carole Lazio, whose comments were particularly helpful.

I owe special thanks to the medical economy division of CREDOC, the Centre de Recherches et de Documentation sur la Consommation (now Credes), especially Dr. Thérèse Lecomte and Ms. Simone Sandier, who made numerous documents available to me. I would also like to thank the staff at the Augustus C. Long Library at the Columbia University Health Sciences Center in New York for their cheerfulness and help during my many long hours spent there.

Thanks to Peggy and Buddy Weiss of the *International Herald Tribune* who helped the book along by hiring me as an editor; jobs such as this, as well as an understanding father, constituted the only financial support outside my advance from the publisher of the project since it (and I) tended to fall between the cracks of established categories of grant eligibility.

Thanks to my European friends whose hospitality helped me to keep the budget low, especially Josephine Markham, Annie Deprez Bouanchaud, Annie Bailleul, Anne Hoffman, Tom and Putzi Lucey, and Darrell Delamaide and Veronika Hass. Thanks to Evelyn Jacobs for her help on the focus. Thanks to my sister Cheryl for setting an example that challenged me to follow. And thanks to all my friends who refrained from asking, "Aren't you ever going to finish that book?"

Index

Abel-Smith, Brian, 106
Abrahams, Robert, 143
Acar, Jacques, 42, 68
Ackerknecht, Erwin, H., 92
Adams, Henry, 108
Aesthetics, 53–55
Age structures, 18
AIDS, xii
    AZT and, xvi
    French treatment of, xvii, 39, 164n
Alcohol
    homeopathy and, 99
    pregnancy and, 146–47
Allergies, 69
Allopathic medicine, 98
Alternative therapies, 19, 65, 77, 97
American College of Radiology, xix
American Heart Association, 134–35
American medicine, See United States
Anemia, 60, 146, 167n
Anesthesiology, 45, 115
Angina pectoris, 23
Antacids, 158n
Anthroposophic medicine, 97–98
Antibiotics, 92–94, 118. See also Drugs
    in France, 62, 66
    lactobacillus prescribed while taking, 41–42
    in United States, 134–35, 144
    in West Germany, 92–94
Antibodies, 169n
Antidepressants, 113–14

Appetite, lack of, 56
Armand, Jean-Pierre, 53
Aromatherapy, 62, 65. See also "Fringe medicine"
Aron-Brunetière, R., 68
Artificial hearts, 152
Austria, 23, 33
Authoritarianism of physicians, 76
Autointoxication, 117

Bad Wörishofen (spa), 91
Balance, in West German medicine, 89–90
Baldness clinic, French, 44–45
Ball, Mark, 64, 76, 84, 87, 90, 93, 96
Bartling, William, 133
Barzini, Luigi, 119, 131
Baum, Michael, 102, 109
Beauté et la Médicine, La (Aron-Brunetière), 68
Béclère, Claude, 47
Belgium, 33
Beller, Fritz, 32–33
Benhamou, Jean-Pierre, 57, 136
Béraud, Claude, 57–59
Bernard, Claude, 39
Besançon, François, 72
Bettelheim, Bruno, 151
Bile ducts, 58–59
Birth. See Childbirth
Birth control. See Contraception
Birth rates, 47–50

Lynn Payer is the author of *How to Avoid a Hysterectomy* and *Disease Mongers: How Doctors, Drug Companies and Insurers Are Making You Feel Sick*. She has taught medical writing at New York University, Columbia University, and Indiana University. She is also the editor of *Medicine and Culture Update: A Newsletter on International Health Differences, Outcomes, and Values*.